HEALING THROUGH TIME

The Complete Guide to Reincarnation and Past Life Regression

WRITTEN BY:

LAUREL PHELAN

authorHOUSE®

AuthorHouse™
1663 Liberty Drive
Bloomington, IN 47403
www.authorhouse.com
Phone: 1-800-839-8640

First published by AuthorHouse   3/17/2010

ISBN: 978-1-4490-8532-2 (e)
ISBN: 978-1-4490-8531-5 (sc)

Printed in the United States of America
Bloomington, Indiana

This book is printed on acid-free paper.

TABLE OF CONTENTS

AUTHOR'S NOTE

OVER THE PAST 25 YEARS, I have worked as a past life regression therapist and have taught reincarnation and regression therapy. I have taken over 2,000 clients through their previous lives and have experienced approximately 50 of my own. This book is the result of those experiences.

From the beginning, I recognized that there was a great importance to understanding reincarnation and looking back on our past lives. Not so as to become focussed on the past, but rather, to better understand the present.

It amazed me how so many of people's problems had no basis in the present but were undoubtedly linked to a previous life experience. I began working with people who had difficulty with anger in their lives or patterns of abuse, either victim or abuser, as well as people with eating disorders and depression. Soon I found more and more people coming to me with everyday problems such as an inability to find love or prosperity, or fears and guilt.

By using self-hypnosis I watched as the subconscious easily opened its memory banks to the roots of problems, most often in a previous life experience.

I realized then the tremendous potential for healing that regression therapy had as well as helping to eliminate hatred, violence and judgement in our society. Once you have experienced yourself as another race or culture you can no longer hate those that are different and once you experience yourself in an impoverished or downtrodden life you no longer judge. More importantly, once you remember that you chose that life, then no longer can you blame anyone else for it.

CHAPTER ONE

Introduction

SINCE I WAS A CHILD I had great difficulty sleeping. I slept approximately one to two hours a night. This didn't seem to be a great problem except that as I aged I became more and more tired. I was unable to become involved in normal childhood activities as all I could think about was resting. I used to lie awake at night and think, waiting for daylight to once more surround me.

I never told anyone that I wasn't sleeping, as I didn't know that anything was wrong with me. I never experienced a full night's sleep, so I didn't miss it. My father thought it was wonderful that, unlike my sisters, he never had to wake me up for school in the morning. I was always awake, eyes wide open, to his amazement. As it does, life went on in this manner, until my late teens.

I moved to a small Vancouver apartment with my father who was dying of cancer. I was 18 years old. Since he couldn't sleep from the pain, he would often walk past my room to the bathroom at night. As he did, I would greet him with a groggy, "hello". So began my father's testing of my insomnia.

He would come past my room at various hourly intervals. Again, I would say "hi". Well, needless to say, this was the beginning of a long discussion on sleep. My father recommended I go to the doctor as it certainly wasn't normal to be awake most of the night. That's when I began numerous tests through the medical profession, none of which were of any help. I tried diet changes, exercise programs, bio-feedback, etc.

Then one day two years later, my doctor stated that she could no longer be of assistance and recommended hypnosis therapy. By this time I was becoming desperate. I was so tired during the day I could barely function at work.

I began three months of hypnosis therapy. My therapist, Dr. Lorraine, immediately stated that she could not hypnotize me, as I would not relinquish control. So she taught me self hypnosis.

As we started searching my subconscious, an amazing fear of fire kept showing itself. I thought this was odd because I had never been in, nor seen, a major fire in my lifetime. After three months of weekly sessions, Dr. Lorraine stated that she would like to try something new. She said she would like to try to go further back in time, to before this life. Well I was certainly game for anything by that time, but I never really understood or thought much about what she meant. I was simply tired and fed up.

We began the session as usual and then she directed me further back in time and suddenly, there I was, in Ireland!

Dr. Lorraine asked me to look around and tell her what I saw. An incredible scene began to form in my memory. It was clear and vivid. I described a huge Christmas tree approximately ten feet tall, adorned with tiny candles held in exquisite and ornate brass holders.

I then looked down towards my body and described a long velvety, rust colored skirt and a beige lace high colored blouse, which I was wearing.

Interestingly, it was at this point that I first experienced my logical mind's desire to interfere in the experience. When I noticed the rust colored skirt my mind immediately jumped in and said, "This is impossible, I would never wear that color. I hate that color. This can't be me."

Of course, it wasn't me. I told Dr. Lorraine that my name was Catherine Graham and I lived in this large manor house in Ireland with my father and servants.

I then felt myself turn and look around the room. It was a large room with a vast hearth in one wall. The hearth was glowing with a huge fire and it warmed the room.

I noticed a tiny man sitting in a corner. He was hunched over and seemed to be ill. Immediately I felt my emotions tug at me as I knew this man was my father and I loved him completely.

I explained to my hypnosis therapist that I was the lady of the house and it was Christmas Eve. We were to have a gathering in the house soon and I was very worried about my father, who was extremely ill but who wouldn't go to bed as I requested.

At this time my logical mind interfered again and I found myself trying to ignore it as it shouted at me that this man could not possibly be my father – my father was six foot three and never had a beard in his life. This tiny little man with the red face was nothing like my father.

Naturally, my present day logical mind was having a difficult time understanding how I could possibly emotionally respond to this man, let alone love him so much.

But love him, I did. My heart was full with worry for him as I noticed a woman in a long black dress with a high collar enter the room and question me. She wanted to know if I could come and check on the food, which was to be served when the guests arrived. I told her I would follow her in a moment as I moved towards my father who seemed to be shivering with a chill.

I knelt in front of this man whom I adored and begged him to go to bed. In a gruff voice he replied that he was the man of the house and he would do no such thing. He was intent on greeting his guests and there was nothing I could do to change his mind.

I did manage, however, to get him to agree to move in front of the fire to sit, so that he would be warmer.

I helped him move as I pulled the heavy chair close to the hearth. I settled him there with a blanket over his lap and he seemed content. I looked back at him and felt worry in my heart as I left the room and attended to the servant's questions in the dining room.

After I felt myself discuss the food with the woman in black I returned to the room where I had left my father and felt my heart jump as terror entered every fiber of my being.

I saw before me a horrific scene of my father lying in the hearth with the flames totally engulfing him.

I screamed as I had never screamed before and felt myself rush to him and drag him out of the fire. I beat his clothes with my hands and laid myself over him to stop the flames.

During this period, my emotions were hysterical and I screamed continuously. I could only imagine what Dr. Lorraine must have thought. My logical mind immediately went into a state of frenzy as well as I heard my mind tell me to stop being a fool and stop screaming. I was aware of a battle in my mind, but I felt totally unable to control my emotions.

My logical present day self was telling me to stop crying and screaming over a man I didn't even know, whereas my emotions couldn't help but feel terrified that my father was burning to death.

I soon realized that the man in my lap, my father, was dead. This spurned a deep emotional pain and I wept uncontrollably for about half an hour. I was aware of Dr. Lorraine putting an arm around me to comfort me.

After I finished sobbing, Dr. Lorraine asked me an interesting question. She asked me to call the spirit of my father to come and communicate with me. My logical mind immediately said this was absurd but I did as I was asked and to my surprise I immediately felt his presence there again with me.

Dr. Lorraine asked me to inquire of his spirit if he blamed me for his death, as I had insisted he sit in front of the fire. I immediately received a reply that he did not blame me as he was ready to die and it had nothing to do with me.

Suddenly I was aware of a sense of relief flowing through me, as though a heaviness was lifting from my whole being. I realized that I was carrying this guilt within my own energy field and it had been weighing me down.

Dr. Lorraine then asked me to inquire of the spirit if I would ever meet him again. My logical mind really loved this one and started a continuous blubbering of how ridiculous this whole thing was and nothing made sense anymore. However, the voice of my logical mind was getting fainter and it didn't really distract me anymore.

When I asked the spirit the question, it immediately replied that it would be my father again, in my present life as Laurel.

With that answer a shock wave seemed to rush through my body and I immediately came out of the regression and opened my eyes. I looked at Dr. Lorraine in astonishment and she just nodded her head and smiled.

"Of course", she said. "It all makes sense now." We discussed the regression and I realized that as my father in my present day life, I had spent my entire life protecting him.

When I was a little girl I used to stay awake at night and prowl around the house like a burglar. However, I would only prowl around my father, who slept on the couch in the living room. I remembered how I used to unplug all of the appliances, such as the radio and television, from near to him. I also used to check around him for lit cigarettes as well as checking the ashtrays.

Through my whole life I was always trying to protect my father from fire, yet I never bothered to check anyone else in the house. My father would often comment to me in the morning that the television and radio were unplugged, yet again.

I had spent my entire life up until that point trying to protect my father from going through the same experience of burning to death, because I felt responsible for him burning to death in that previous life.

By the time I had undergone this regression, my present day father had died from cancer almost two years earlier so there was no longer a reason for me to stay awake any longer.

Indeed, that very night I went home and slept for eight straight hours, something I had never, in my entire life, done. I was acutely aware of waking up the next day, which was Sunday, and feeling refreshed and aware that I had actually slept for a long time. It was truly amazing for me and I realized that the regression had healed my insomnia.

When I shared the experience with friends, I immediately received questioning gazes and responses about how vivid an imagination I must have. Needless to say I was hurt and annoyed that no one believed me. But in truth, it didn't really matter. I realized that no one could invalidate my experience. The emotions and visions I experienced as Catherine Graham were so real and intense, there is no way a vivid imagination could have come up with something so powerful.

To this day, almost thirty years later, I can remember every single detail of that regression as if it happened yesterday. A real and powerful memory never fades, whereas imagination does.

CHAPTER TWO

Healing With Regression

ARE YOU FRUSTRATED OR BORED with life? Emotional? Angry? Unhappy? Lonely, fearful or depressed? Then that is enough of a reason for having a past life regression and for learning about reincarnation. To better your present life. Unless you have attained inner peace and love for all, there is always room for growth and discovery. Until you have attained inner peace, you should always keep an open mind to new ideas and be willing to make new discoveries.

Many believe if you have past life regressions, you will become obsessed with the past and forget to live in the present. This is not the case. A regression leads you to a better and more peaceful present life.

When I first learned the regression technique, I too thought that I would do a regression every other day and become obsessed with my past lives. It's interesting however, that this never happens. In fact, the opposite is true. It frees you from the past and allows you a greater wholeness in the present.

People tend to come to me when they already have an obsession or at the very least, a fascination with a time or place. Or if not that, then a problem in their present lives. This is a sign from the past that is trying to get your attention to look back and heal or balance your previous lives in order that you may move onwards and grow.

Someone once asked me during an interview for my book Guinevere, "Isn't it difficult to simply be Laurel now, when you have been Guinevere, and don't you wish you could be her again?" My reply. "Hardly!"

This brought up an interesting theory which I have researched endlessly. When you have been someone in a past life, you don't want to be them again. Even if it was a great life. You've been there and done that and there is no risk that you will become obsessed with that life again. Rather, the opposite is true. You find yourself wanting to heal and move on as soon as possible. It's not that you want to forget about the life, but you very strongly want to be a better you, not some ancient person again.

I also realized something fascinating about obsessions with people from the past. If we are constantly thinking about a person from the past or fantasizing that we were them, there is only a small possibility that we were that person. It is far more likely that we knew that person though and maybe admired or even hated, them.

When we undergo a past life memory, we are freed of our past, not encumbered by it. We are not taking on a load, but releasing one.

A case in point is a lifetime I experienced in France in the early 18th century. For most of my present life I had a fascination with tulle and lace covered hats as well as a habit of draping fabric in a balloon-like manner over tables, around sinks and of course windows. I also collected antiques, especially teacups and pots.

For years my friends would comment on how I had such a Victorian flare for decorating and how I must have lived in 19th century England. However, I knew through my regressions that I had not, in fact, lived in England during that time.

Finally, one evening when I had little to do, I decided to regress myself. I gave my subconscious the instructions that I would go to a nice, pleasant lifetime, if there were any.

To my surprise, I soon found myself in an apartment in Paris, France. The room had billowing fabric draped over the walls, ceiling and of course, everything in the room. I knew my name and my place of work, which was a shop that I owned at 52 rue de la Seine, Paris, France.

Upon going to the shop in the regression, I found that it was filled with gorgeous, overly fancy, hats made of tulle, lace and large feathers. I discovered that I designed hats, and specialized in large funeral hats with black lace overhangs.

After the regression I looked around my home and realized where my decorating habits originated. Interestingly, however, as soon as I came out of the regression, my tastes immediately changed. I found that I no longer wanted the lace and billowing fabric everywhere. The reason being – I was now complete with that time period. I needed to return to that lifetime in order to remember my creative side as well as my flare for decorating. However, now I wanted to change my décor immediately.

When we journey into our past life memories, we do not become fascinated with that time. Instead, we drop the fascination which we have probably already had.

People have many reasons for wanting a past life regression, including simple curiosity. But the most common reason is because something is not working in their present life or they have a specific problem which is plaguing them.

Past life regression can help problems ranging from depression, eating disorders, anger, lack of self worth to fears and phobias as well as physical disorders. The list is endless.

This is not to say that past life regression is a cure all. It certainly is not. But it can assist us in finding the causes to our current day problems and illnesses. It offers a way to release the cause and then allow the healing to take place.

This works in a most simplistic way. A present day issue such as fear for instance, will have a cause somewhere in our past.

It is natural to say that if we have a problem it has a cause. Regression offers a window to find that cause and then to release the emotion surrounding it, thereby freeing us from the problem.

Not all causes to present problems are in a past life, however, and this is why regression can be used to find causes to problems in our present life as well.

Regression is simply a tool to enter the subconscious memory, which knows no bounds of time.

The key to finding the cause of the present day problem is to direct the subconscious to finding the cause, where ever it may be. It may sound difficult, but it isn't. A simple suggestion from the regression therapist sends the subconscious on a search, just like a computer. It seeks out and finds the memory which relates to the present day problem.

Then the memory is brought to the forefront and the person re-experiences the cause to the problem.

In order to heal with past life regression, it is necessary, however, not just to visually see the past memory, but to re-experience it. In other words, to feel yourself within the past life body or childhood body, not to see it from a distance.

Present day problems are caused by emotions from our previous lives which have not been expressed and healed. As is still common today, we are taught to suppress our feelings and to stuff our emotions deep inside until we no longer feel them.

Unfortunately, the energy within these emotions does not go away, it is still within our vast energy field, it has simply been hidden. This emotional energy stays with us and most often, irritates our lives in some way until we release it and heal our past. So no matter how much we try to stuff our feelings, they aren't going to go away.

Some of the emotional experiences that we move through in our everyday lives are quite small and we naturally, through the course of everyday living, emit them and heal. However, some of the more intense emotions are not healed through everyday living and it is these that we carry from lifetime to lifetime until we finally allow them to be released and healed. Some people feel that simply expressing emotions continually will free them from all past life emotional baggage. This is not true. We must also learn from the experience as well.

CHAPTER THREE

Why We Are Here

As a spirit, before we even come into the body, we recognize that the whole experience of humanhood is one of illusion in order to learn about suffering and separation in order to eventually remember that we are complete love.

If we were simply going to create a planet filled with joy and bliss, there really would be no point to the experiment at all, would there?

Look around our planet and you will see that throughout history it has been a planet of barbarism and cruelty with a smidgen of joy and love thrown in just to keep us going. It's certainly not a paradise and not a place of peace. It's a place of anger, struggle and suffering, and yet people continually try to convince themselves that this experience of life is divine and wonderful. Look again, and this time be honest. When, throughout history, has the human race experienced bliss and unity, let alone complete love and joy? It hasn't. Rather, it's been a place dominated by war and conflict, ego and fear.

It's a planet where we watch children suffer and writhe in pain and yet we continue to believe it is a paradise that God created. We also continue to convince ourselves that somehow children suffering is God's divine plan and we must simply accept that God knows more than we do.

Don't get me wrong, I am not a cynical person. Far from it. But I do realize that it's time that we looked at the truth about this planet. People keep expecting that some divine being is going to come down to the planet and then everything will be wonderful again. Again?! When was it ever wonderful?

Certainly the Christian belief that their savior, Jesus, will return is something of a fantasy. When he was here the first time, they persecuted him and murdered him. Why would today be any different?

No matter what wonderful teachers come to the planet to teach us to love, it is inherent within people to be cruel, angry and egomaniacal. Why? Because that's a part of their evolutionary path and until they evolve into very old souls, they are not going to change and neither is the mass majority of people on the planet.

It amazes me to find people continually postponing their own responsibility because they are waiting for someone to come and save them or at the very least, to fix everything on the planet. It certainly has never happened before and there is no reason to believe that it's going to happen now.

The responsibility, therefore, for our happiness, is not in the hands of someone else, but in our own hands, where it has always been and it is time to begin changing ourselves from within rather than waiting for someone else to do it for us, or waiting for everyone in the world to somehow all change at the same time.

The planet was created as a place to experience separateness. Period. Through that separateness we experience many other facets of humanness, including pain, aloneness and greed. The list is endless. We also experience moments of love, joy and peace.

Ultimately, however, we will come to remember that the experience of humanness is an illusion, as is the planet. Science has already shown us that we are not solid, as we seem to look. We are atoms and quantum energy, nothing more. Even the walls and rocks are energy moving at different frequencies which make them look and feel more solid to us. But they aren't solid. Therefore, the visual experience of the planet is illusory.

If bodies are not solid and walls are actually moving, vibrating energy, as is the earth beneath our feet, then all that we have come to believe is reality, is not. So then it's time to look further into understanding of what and who we really are.

Science tells us that everything on the planet, including our bodies, is energy. Therefore, we are all united and linked, right? Energy doesn't differentiate from itself. There isn't good energy and bad energy. There is simply energy, and if we are energy, which we are, then we are not really cruel and mean, or funny or boring, or even good looking or ugly.

We are the energy within the cell which then creates a body and a brain. By creating a blueprint before we are born, we also create an ego/personality to be used within the body in order to engage in the illusion of humanness. Once we leave the illusion, through death, we carry the memory of the personality/ego with us, but we are no longer attached to it as the ego/personality is only used whilst in the body. There is no reason for it outside of the body. We can carry the memories because we take the energy with us.

So we are not bodies and not really separate from each other, but rather, we are here to undertake a growth experience of finding out who we are by separating from our source. That source is loving, infinite energy.

To say that energy has no wisdom, I feel is not accurate. Wisdom is not thought or knowledge, it is awareness of truth. To say that energy has no understanding of love is also not accurate. This awareness can only be fully understood by experiencing it yourself, because once you leave the body and the ego/personality and stripped yourself of the illusionary qualities of the planet, including desire, personality traits, greed, etc., there is something left, and that something never leaves. It is love. A love so profound and fulfilling that it eliminates all emptiness and aloneness.

This is the love that we have left behind when we took on a body and when we return to it after we've completed with all of our lives, we remember that it is truth.

Still, when we have taken on a commitment to move through the illusionary experiences of lives on this planet, we have chosen separateness, not because we did not experience divine love from our source, the universal energy, but we did not know that we, if separate, were love as well.

In other words, picture a large formation of loving, brilliantly lit energy, pulsing infinitely in space. There is unity and oneness, yet small sparks of energy pull apart in order to experience separateness. This separate and aware energy, which has conscious awareness, but not ego/mind or personality, still feels at one with the universal energy and does not fully know if the love it is experiencing is from the universal energy or from within itself.

So these energy sparks choose to be a part of an experiment with masses of other energy sparks on the same quest, and create a planet where true separateness will be experienced. Then they will undergo a series of illusions of great hardship in order to discover if, even through the worst illusion of aloneness, they are a part of the universe and are love themselves, or if the universal energy is like a God-force and supreme to them.

It's almost the same as when you are in a large group or organization where everyone is dedicated to the same thing. It can be hard to know where you fit in or if you matter. Can the group get along without you, or are you really a necessary and vital part of it? Does the group have one supreme being running the show, or are we all equal and the sum of all of us are what makes it run. Only by separating from the universal energy source can we know if we are truly, loving energy as well, or if we are simply being held in it and it is something outside of us.

The process of enlightenment is one of discovering that the love we had experienced as an energy formation while out of the body is not outside of us, but it is in the core of our energy, it is who we are as well. The combined loving energy of all is united and therefore, creates a greater loving force, or divine universal energy. It is not that a supreme being is the only one who loves and we are simply blessed by being given that love.

This is what we are here to learn, or as I prefer, to remember. That we are love itself, not that we can be loving, but we are love. It is within our core, it is who we are. We are love energy, not a body or personality or even an energy force with no purpose.

Our purpose is to find that inner love and then we will return to the universal loving energy source and complete with this cycle of reincarnations and the illusion of separateness. Then the universal energy is greater because our loving energy enhances it as we are a necessary part of it.

Much of the difficulty that people have with their lives is the feeling of uselessness and not really being a necessary part of existence.

I have often felt that this is why the movie, "It's a Wonderful Life", has such impact to this day on people. Because we want to know that we are needed and not useless.

Only by finding our inner love, however, do we eventually come to realize that we are not only necessary, but an integral part of the universal energy force.

Universal energy is the sum of all of us and when we truly remember this, not intellectually, by reading about it, but inwardly, by knowing, we reach enlightenment. Enlightenment is, after all, remembering the light within.

CHAPTER FOUR

What Is Reincarnation?

To UNDERSTAND REINCARNATION IS TO understand the basic principles of life. If you look around your environment, you will notice that everything has cycles of life, death and rebirth. The flowers and trees are born and as they move through the seasons they die and again are reborn in the spring. Nature is the fundamental basis of all life and we are a part of nature. The cycles of life and death move in circles, as does all energy. We are also made up of energy and as such, are no different than the rest of the world around us, including nature.

Reincarnation is the cycle of death and rebirth for the purpose of growth and evolvement. Through my own experiences and those of my clients, I have come to understand that this circle is not meaningless by any means.

When I took people through their previous lives and death experiences, I would ask them some standard questions. The most important one being, "Why are you here?" The responses were always greatly similar or identical in over 2,000 cases.

They would answer that they had separated from Light, their source, to come into human form to find love through different experiences. When they first separated from the universal light or energy, as some chose to call it, their own energy was very small. As they grew and evolved through many lives and life experiences, their light or energy grew until they would ultimately return from whence they came and no longer enter a body again. This process is often called Enlightenment.

Enlightenment is when our energy has experienced all it can possibly experience in the human form and can no longer contain its energy within the confines of a body. It then rejoins the universal light, bringing with it more energy and thus, more light and love.

How does energy grow? Love. Through numerous lives we grow and experience, often through adversity and pain, and eventually find love in all that is around us. It is through this giving and receiving of love that we ultimately find enlightenment or bliss, and no longer need to continue the circle of death and rebirth.

CHAPTER FIVE

Where Did It All Begin And Where Does It End

IT BEGAN WITH ENERGY. LIGHT is energy and vice versa. Energy has always existed and always will. Science has proven that humans are made of energy. They have also proven that you cannot destroy energy. Therefore, when we die something must happen to that energy. Where does it go? Obviously it doesn't die. This is where physics ends and metaphysics takes over. We come to a point where we must begin to trust our intuition and seek the answers that lie in our memories.

Most ancient civilizations believed in reincarnation because they felt more at one with nature. As we have become "civilized" (and sometimes this can be questioned), we have separated ourselves from nature and spirituality and become individualized, or as I prefer, ego-ized.

Mechanical and logical thinking has convinced us that reincarnation does not exist. Why? Because reincarnation has nothing to do with logic. It cannot be proven to the satisfaction of the logical mind, so most people feel there is no point in trying. What is wiser to remember is that there are other things that cannot be proven by logic either, namely "love".

No scientist can prove love, yet we know it exists. How? By feeling.

Feeling flows through the right side of the brain. The intuitive and knowing self. Logic and intellect (ego) come through the left side of the brain. They seldom meet with comfort. When there is an intuitive or emotional experience there is often judgement about that experience.

When a person moves from day to day living, which is usually existing through the left brain, into their right brain, there is an immediate struggle for the logical self or ego to regain control. The logical part of our mind doesn't like to be out of control. Unfortunately what often happens is the logical self invalidates our intuitive or emotional experiences.

As all beings do, we begin as energy. We spark from the universal light or god force, if you prefer, and form an individual, yet tiny, light force. During that process we do not become abandoned in any way, nor do we lose our connection with the universal light. It is who we are. It is the source from whence we came. It is our very essence.

Once on our own, we begin to move through the evolutionary process of growth. Beginning as a tiny form of life we then start to experience life on our planet.

In our first forms of life we don't experience as much of a separate feeling as we do later in human form when we take on ego, but rather experience more of a oneness with creation. Rather than thought there is feeling and instinct. We may very easily experience many lives moving through the chain of existence, i.e. the plant kingdom and the animal kingdom.

When we have fully experienced all there is on the above levels, it is time to move onward, to humanness.

CHAPTER SIX

Ego

WITH THE HUMAN FORM COMES extra baggage, namely the ego. Ego is, in its simplest form, intellect or logical and mechanical thinking. Intellect/ Ego longs to control and place all experiences into a neat little logical package. It does not understand love and intuition, therefore it is the human's greatest challenge to enlightenment.

Ego keeps us firmly entrenched in the reincarnation circle and the belief that we are separate from the whole and, therefore, causes us to become trapped in thought forms and logic rather than feeling and intuition.

To end the reincarnation circle, one must first understand the ego and the desire it has to keep us feeling separate and alone. Reincarnation teaches us to remember that we are not separate nor are we alone. We are simply spirit energy temporarily encased in the human body, or costume, as I like to call it.

Ego keeps us stuck in survival mode and seeking validation outside of ourselves because we have forgotten that we are spirit and, in fact, one with all of existence.

Ego works with logic and mechanical thinking and continually creates a feeling of insecurity in our lives, which further creates a lifelong struggle for security. Security in relationships, money, etc.

If you look around you in the world you will see how much focus is on the quest for financial and emotional security. This is not surprising because the majority of the population of the planet is ego based and has completely forgotten that they are a vibrating spiritual energy within. They have forgotten that they took on the ego in order to learn about aloneness and separateness and eventually return to wholeness, and have come to believe that they are, in fact, the ego or personality. How often do you hear the statement, "He bruised his ego" or "It was a blow to his ego"?

The ego has been elevated to God status in our world and it needs to be brought back in line. It does not help our spiritual path to focus our entire lives on strengthening the ego, rather we should be looking at how to dissolve it. It is a tool that has become the master and people the willing servants to its continual quest for materiality/greatness and outer validation.

So often I have come across people who continually ask the question, "How do I look", or "What should I do?" They have forgotten who they are within and are continually asking others, who have also forgotten, to tell them who they are and if they are of worth.

When you continually look to others to validate you or your decisions, you are disempowering yourself and stating to the universe that you do not know who you are and maybe some complete stranger or at best, a relative, does.

Do you really think your mate or family member knows who you are, when you don't even know yourself? In truth, you are the only one who can validate who you are and only by looking within and finding it yourself, not by asking someone else. Because the ego has created this illusion of separateness and aloneness, you have forgotten self and are constantly relying on someone else to help you discover yourself, when, in fact, those people are in the same boat as you and have no idea who they are either.

The ego is of great importance in understanding the cycles of death and rebirth or reincarnation because it is this illusion of separateness that keeps us continually coming back into body after body. By looking at our past lives, we discover that we are not bodies and egos or personalities at all, but spirits moving through different bodies in order to evolve to pure love once again and to enhance our energy.

Remembering our past lives disconnects us from the illusory game of the ego and helps us to know and feel our truth, the spiritual self, not the false egos and personalities.

When you move through various lives and experience yourself as different personalities in different cultures and races, not to mention different sexes, you understand that you are not an ego or personality, or even a body. You are the energy that empowers the cell, which empowers the body, brain and ego/personality.

One of the reasons to move through our past lives and remember these experiences is to detach from the ego and find our true selves. In order to find our spiritual path, the ego must become the tool once again, not the master, and moving into our past lives gives us the ability to distance ourselves from it and to have a greater understanding of how it has manipulated our lives and kept us in the dark about our truth and spirituality.

In the workshops I teach called "The Path To Enlightenment", I help people to recognize the ego through various exercises. As most people are unable to recognize the subtleties of the ego and have become focussed on the obvious ego. The obvious ego being when someone is continually praising themselves to others and is absolutely fascinated with his outer appearance or achievements.

This form of ego expression is easily identified but there are far more subtle expressions that you need to be able to recognize in order to be able to drop them. For instance the desire to acquire knowledge and titles or the fascination with your name.

Names and titles are all false layers that you build around you in order to enhance the illusion. This is a very common ego expression and our world greatly encourages it.

Since childhood you are taught to acquire knowledge and to become someone or something. You begin to introduce yourself to others by a title or occupation. How often have you responded to someone by saying, "I am a nurse, doctor, lawyer, secretary, housewife, janitor, or whatever"? You state that you are your occupation, when in fact, your occupation is just something you do. It is not who you are.

When you place letters at the end of your name you believe you are enhancing yourself, but in actuality you are placing yourself in a box, and the box is called the ego. By giving yourself a title or identifying greatly with your name you are actually limiting yourself immensely.

You are a spirit, and a spirit is limitless. You are far more divine than any degree, title, or personality. No matter how much knowledge you acquire you are still a spirit within, just like everyone else.

I found it interesting many years ago when I was invited to attend a meeting of the Mensa Society in Canada. The Mensa are a group of people who have created an organization based on their high I.Q.'s. They tend to dedicate themselves to acquiring knowledge. When sitting and discussing life with them, however, I found it fascinating that most of them had very little common sense when it came to life experiences, and the ones that I spoke to were so wrapped up in their intellects that they had little feeling and certainly a very small, if not completely absent, capacity for intuition.

In their ego's desire to proclaim their vast intelligence, they had placed themselves in a box where only knowledge was allowed. There was no room for wisdom and certainly none for intuition or emotion.

In my research over the last twenty-five years, I have focussed on the limitations that the group mind places on people. We are taught from youth to be joiners, to get involved with groups and organizations. Unfortunately, most groups and organizations have leaders and rules, or at the least, structure. These rules and structures are not empowering to people, as they would have you believe, but rather, limiting to people.

In our society we are taught to enhance the outer by building layer upon layer of stuff. Namely, knowledge, titles, becoming involved in an organization or group, or even a religion. It gives people the illusion that they are special because they have a title or because they are a part of some institution or group.

These are ego layers that you continually build lifetime after lifetime and yet, the real question should be: are these groups, titles, names, etc., truly fulfilling you?

When I met with the Mensa group, I noticed most people had at least one degree under their belt and were often working on another one, ultimately seeking a Ph.D., which seemed the top goal. Yet when I talked privately with some of them about their personal lives and happiness, it seemed almost foreign to them. I questioned them on what was enough for them. Those that had their Ph.D.'s still found themselves seeking more and more. Those that had accomplished fantastic feats of intelligence and even inventions were still empty inside.

You will notice the same feelings with people who have amassed great wealth. Are they at peace and truly happy within themselves? No, they are not. They continually seek more, because when one desire of ego's is fulfilled then emptiness sets in again and they need another desire or goal to work towards. This is the key to understanding the ego. It continually causes you to focus on the future and goals. You see, the ego can never be satisfied. If you experience peace and satisfaction in the moment, then there is no ego, ego dissolves.

The difficulty, however, is that ego has been encouraged by society and your teachings to continually keep you focussed on the future and seeking more and more. Either you seek money or knowledge or adventure, but there is always something.

The ego cannot rest in the moment, because when you allow yourself to be fully accepting in the moment without desiring and projecting into the future, then ego is no longer there, and then you experience peace and spirituality. One of the things I have noticed in taking many people through their past lives is that they realize that the continual quest for exterior sources of pleasure and ego enhancement does not lead to peace and happiness, rather, it leads to more quests and a greater ego.

I would often guide people into their most powerful lives where they found themselves stuck in a never ending search for even more power, even when they were a ruler or leader. Look at Napoleon or Caesar, do you think they were satisfied? Hardly. In fact, the greater the outer power one accumulates, the more one wants. The ego has become so strong, that the spirit within is completely hidden by the great mask around it. The ego is in control, not you, the spirit.

In journeying into your past lives, I would encourage you to remember those lives where you had great wealth, knowledge or outer power. By re-experiencing them you will find it easier to detach from ego in your present life and begin the journey to finding your true self, the spirit within.

Remember that the ego also creates the illusion of separateness and aloneness. How can you be alone, you are a spirit and a part of all spirit energy in the universe. You are not separate. Energy is not different from other energy, but in taking on a body and an ego/intellect, you have taken on a mask which convinces you that you are separate. In order to find your wholeness again and your true self, you must take off the mask and look inside for your self, not outside, which is what the ego is continually doing.

The ego keeps you seeking new careers or identities and you continually hope that a new identity or job or new home will make you happy within.

No outside experience, job or change in your personality or relationship can bring you to inner wholeness and peace. Only by stripping away the false layers of ego and looking inside, through meditation and acceptance of the present moment, will you be able to find your true self and with that finding, reconnect to all that is, universal energy and love.

One key to dissolving ego is silence, stillness and sacredness.

Create silence in your life and your mind by sitting and allowing a sacredness to bubble up from within you. By releasing the pursuit of happiness and accepting yourself as a spirit in this moment, without projecting into the future, you allow yourself to move deeper into the core of your being where ego does not exist – but true happiness does.

Under the many layers of false masks and ego identifications there sits a divine spirit energy that has been there all along. You do not need to seek your spirit self, but to uncover it, for it has always been there and always will be there. Remember, the mask/ego covers your spirit, but the spirit still remains within.

CHAPTER SEVEN

Love

IT'S IMPORTANT TO ACCEPT THAT love from those around us can never truly fulfill the emptiness inside. What we seek is ourselves, or the remembrance of ourselves.

Because ego creates forgetfulness that we are spirits and connected to all that is around us, it also creates a constant need for that emptiness to be filled. So we seek it from others. But the true way to filling the emptiness is by remembering that we are spirits, not bodies or personalities, and we are not separate as ego would like us to believe, but rather, one with everyone and everything that exists.

When we remember our past lives and understand reincarnation, we begin a process of filling the emptiness in our hearts as we become more connected to those around us. There is no longer a need for others to love us because we have never been separate, we simply forgot who we were.

The more you remember that you are a spirit, the more whole and loved you feel.

The only way to disempower the ego is to move into the heart and love. With true, unconditional love, there cannot be ego. Intellect does not understand love, because love is intuitive and emotional, not logical. Therefore, when true love is experienced, ego dissolves.

I was walking with a friend one day in the woods and he would regularly say "hello", to whoever passed us by. Most often people would reply, "hello", in return but on the odd occasion the person would not only ignore my friend's hello, but look away as if pretending not to have heard him. This used to make my friend quite upset and he would then comment on how rude that person was. As we continued on our walk, I noticed that he did not say hello to the next person that walked by. I asked him why not and he replied, "What's the point?"

The point was that he was giving his love in the form of a hello on a conditional basis: that the person return that love. If they didn't return it, then he would withhold his love from then on.

I often noticed this with people afterwards. They thought they were wonderful human beings by offering a gesture of love through their hello or maybe a wave or greeting. The ego felt great, especially if someone returned the gesture, then the ego felt more special because they had given something to make that person's day nicer. But that is not unconditional love. It is ego based, conditional love.

It shouldn't matter whether someone receives your love or whether or not they return it. If you give, do so without requiring recognition for it. The true giver of love expects nothing in return, not even an acknowledgement.

CHAPTER EIGHT

Judgement

ANOTHER GAME THE EGO LIKES to play is called judgement. We are forever judging others or criticizing them in some way. This empowers the ego and creates a greater sense of individuality and unfortunately aloneness. The more you judge, the more alone you become.

Reincarnation teaches us that judgement is pointless. For you have been, or will become, those whom you judge. You experience all forms of costumes or bodies through the reincarnation cycle. Fat ones, thin ones, tall ones and short ones. You experience being deformed and ugly as well as beautiful and physically superb. You have been a beggar and a rich person, a smart and a simple one. So you see, judging another is only showing lack of understanding. Which is why it is so important to re-experience your past lives.

By feeling yourself in the body of another race or maybe a physically deformed person, you create empathy for all those around you because you have been there and you begin to recognize that everyone is merely a spirit in a costume.

When you go to a costume party you do not believe that the people inside are really the characters they are dressed as, and so you should not believe spirits are the bodies or personalities they are enclosed in.

A personality is another form of ego. Like a mask that is covering the true self, the spirit.

We need to look beyond the mask and the body and see that the spirits or energy inside us are all the same, identical in every way. When you recognize this, you eliminate judgement and open up a whole new world of love for yourself.

Our society is rife with judgement. We judge each other's race, religion, sex. Even countries and cities. We are taught to judge since childhood. Do you remember thinking that your city was better than another city? Or your country as better than other countries? Even that your school was better than other schools?

When we see someone walking by, we judge their bodies and anything else we can think of because we've been taught that we are individual and "different". But we're not.

For this reason, I feel learning about reincarnation is so important because it absolutely eliminates hatred and judgement by taking away the belief that we are "different" from each other.

I once took a client into a past life who had been rather racist again Orientals and chauvinistic to women. He soon found himself in a rice paddy in China as a woman giving birth. This totally shifted his consciousness. After the regression he became compassionate and understanding to both Orientals and women.

CHAPTER NINE

Beliefs And Christianity

I WAS FASCINATED TO LEARN that most religions, including Christianity, in the beginning, believed in reincarnation. Through my studies of various religions, I have often found it interesting that the teachings of reincarnation did not interfere with their religious beliefs. It is really only Christianity and Judaism that disagree with reincarnation and in fact, Christianity actually does agree with it. That is if you journey back to the original teachings. It is even well documented in the Indian Sanskrit documents of a period of two years that Jesus spent in India studying, among other things, reincarnation.

What seemed to have happened was, in the sixth century, Roman Christian leaders under the influence of Emperor Justinian, felt it necessary to eradicate references about reincarnation from their religious documents. Why was that? Well, to begin with, it was a way of controlling people.

First it's important to look at the time when the changes in the documents were taking place. For Christianity it was the sixth century. Most of the religious scriptures up to that time spoke about reincarnation. The Gnostic Gospel to this day speaks of "The soul spilling from one body into another".

People who understood reincarnation tended to be free thinkers and unwilling to be controlled by leaders or by fear.

In that time period, fear was the way for most leaders to rule and if their subjects were too independent they were a threat to the community. So began the slow destruction of the teachings of reincarnation.

Christians have often argued to me that reincarnation goes against Christianity. "Does it really?" was my reply. Well, let's look at that.

Reincarnation teaches us that we are all equal to each other. It also teaches us to love and accept everyone, not just those with the same beliefs. Reincarnation eliminates racism and greed and cruelty, as we learn that we will have to balance it in our future through karma. Reincarnation teaches us to be compassionate, accepting and loving. It teaches us to find our truth through humbly looking within and finding the light of the universe within ourselves, not from worshipping someone else's experience.

Yes, maybe they were right, maybe reincarnation does go against Christianity, which teaches us to fear God.

Obviously a God that must be feared cannot be a loving, compassionate and forgiving God. Religion constantly contradicts itself with the statements of a total loving God and then a God that must be feared.

Christianity also teaches us not to accept our fellow man as they are, but to change him and accept him as our equal only if he becomes a Christian. Otherwise he is considered a heathen and unworthy of God.

Christians have been known to be notorious, as have many other religions over the ages, at torturing and murdering those that do not convert and accept their ways. This is hardly loving and compassionate acceptance. It is control and domination through the use of force and fear.

Often, as a child growing up in a Catholic family, I found myself frustrated when we went to church on Sunday. The priest would spew his sermon with great verve and words that went right over my head. One day I decided I had had enough and raised my arm to ask a question, as I had been taught to do in school. Well, my mother was not impressed and quickly pulled my arm back down. She gave me a stern look and told me to be still.

I learned something profound that day, although the implications never truly took hold until I became an adult.

In school I was encouraged to raise my hand and ask questions, which meant that I was curious and a good learner. In church, raising my hand meant that I was a troublemaker.

For a long time I wondered why we were not allowed to question anything that the church said, yet we were encouraged to question the teacher in school. Weren't the priests our teachers too? Weren't we being taught religion? We certainly weren't born with it. Why were we being told to blindly accept without question when it came to religion and to challenge when it came to other teachings?

It was obvious to me as I grew that when we question our teachers in school, it promotes growth and change and children learn to expand their ideas beyond what their parents were taught regarding science, physics, technology, etc.

With religion, however, we were taught never to question, because questioning promotes growth and change and religions don't tolerate growth and change.

If religions were discussed and debated rather than blindly accepted, then most of them would no longer be a part of our lives, as we would have outgrown them and changed. But if you look back in history, religious leaders were also politicians and that leads us to a most important discovery.

Politicians and religious leaders wanted all the power and so began to punish people who questioned any religious or political belief or doctrine. Since the Roman times, people have been persecuted and murdered for challenging the religious beliefs of the day. Actually even during Egyptian times as well.

It didn't take people long to discover that challenging religious teachings meant death and so this attitude that it is better to follow without questioning began to be taught from parent to child from ancient times. It was much safer never to question.

Prior to the Roman teachings, the Greek culture thrived in its philosophical discussions and is often credited with being the first free thinking society and the first civilized society.

During the height of the Greek culture, philosophers and the general public openly discussed and challenged spiritual, mental and scientific concepts and beliefs. This created a great society of advanced awareness, although still mostly limited to discussing rather than experiencing. It was the beginning of true freedom of thought and speech, which unfortunately did not last.

What we should learn from our history is that following another's beliefs has not led us to peace or enlightenment, nor bliss within ourselves.

It is time to take the power back and find our truth about death and spirituality, rather than just discussing and fantasizing about it or taking someone else's word for it.

Then the question arises – How? How do you find out for yourself? You can't die and come back and then say, now I know! Or can you? That's where past life regression comes in.

One thing I have learned in my spiritual search is that religion and spirituality are not the same thing. Religion is organized. It is based on following someone else's experience and worshipping someone else's experience. Spirituality, on the other hand, is about finding your own spiritual experience and inner truth. Spirituality is awakening an inner wisdom, whereas religion is knowledge acquired from an outside source.

Religion creates rules and structure, whereas through the spiritual quest, one awakens inner morals and truths and lives in love and peace.

With religion people need to be told what to do because they have not experienced their own truth and spiritual self.

With a spiritual path, one finds their own inner self and through self love, loves others and respects life and all beings.

CHAPTER TEN

Choice

THIS CHAPTER WILL PROBABLY BE the one that you will have the most difficulty with accepting. I have found through the years that people tend to find the teachings of choice the most difficult to embrace, at first. This is usually because of their upbringing, where they were taught that they were a victim.

People like to believe that they choose the positive experiences in their lives but not the negative ones, or as has become very popular in our society, to blame someone else for our problems.

Let's face it, no one wants to believe they were a murderer or war monger in the past. We all want to believe we were wonderful, loving, and generous people, heroes and heroines in our society, admired by all. Well that would be wonderful, but who would play the other parts, and as we have seen throughout history, people have been brutal and barbarous and still are.

Life here on the planet is like a great big costume drama. Some play the bad guys and some the good guys. Then we reverse roles and try it again. Ultimately, we remember that the whole thing is an illusion and we return to remembering that we are spirits trying to find love through the complexities of the costume party.

We like to judge the bad guys and say they are not like us but we must remember that they are like us, in fact exactly like us. They too have forgotten that they are spirits and have become stuck in the personality and ego and the costume or body.

In so doing, we all experience anger, violence and suffering. The whole range of emotions in fact. It is all part of the experience.

What we learn from understanding reincarnation is that there is a way out of the ignorance of violence and suffering. That is by remembering that it is a costume drama and we are not the bodies and personalities but rather, the spiritual energy inside.

Forgetfulness has created such deep suffering on our planet and it shows no signs of ending. I have often heard of people calling ancient civilizations brutal or uncivilized in their manner of treating people through sacrifice, etc. What I find interesting is that they believe we as a civilization have changed. In actuality we are still the same, no better than barbarians. We still murder and then judge the murderer and murder him in return. We are still quick to judge and have retribution. It is a cycle of ignorance which the ego and personality creates by telling us that we are individual.

The choices we make in life are not conscious, but spiritual, in unison with our higher selves. As a whole spirit before birth, we choose what our next lifetime is going to be for. In other words, which experience or lesson is to be undertaken in our evolutionary path.

This is not forced upon us by a hierarchy of spirits but is chosen by ourselves. We then choose our parents. In doing this, we look at the people that will most be able to help us in our next learning experience. Sometimes we will need to wait until the appropriate parents come together or the appropriate world events come together.

For instance, we might be choosing to experience a war or an event involving a mass amount of people and would need to wait for such events to come closer to together. Sometimes we will wait to experience life with a certain spirit that we have a karma with and as such would need to wait for them to be in a body.

As a spirit you are not alone or isolated but connected to other spirit energy in the astral realm as well as being guided by energies that no longer move through the process of reincarnation. This is where you will choose to create an agreement with another spirit's higher self to undergo some experience together, so that you both may learn and evolve.

If another spirit is already embodied and you want to undertake an experience with them then one wonders, how can you make an agreement with someone who is already in a body and therefore forgets that they are a spirit and cannot hear you?

Before coming into the body your energy is whole. Imagine a circle of energy. When you enter the body, half of that energy or circle enters and half stays on the astral realm, which is dimension of energy surrounding us. That half is what is most often called your "higher self". This higher energy has full understanding of your chosen path while the energy that takes on the body and personality has forgotten. Therefore, your higher self is always making choices, probably with other higher selves or spirits not yet in a body. Your higher self does not make the choices based on what your ego wants but rather, what is of the highest good for you in learning your lessons for the lifetime.

So it is not a matter of conscious choice in the body/mind, but higher self's choice. Therefore, it is quite important to learn to spiritually connect with your higher self in order to understand what your path is and enable you to work together, rather than having your conscious self in ignorance and feeling like a victim rather than a creator.

No matter how many success courses or positive thoughts you think, if you are not conscious of your spiritual self you will often feel like a victim of circumstance. When you become connected spiritually to your higher self, then you recognize that you actually have conscious power to make choices and changes in your path. You begin to work with your higher self rather than allowing higher self to make all the choices for you.

Think of your body as a vehicle, a car for instance. In general most of us are sitting in the back seat of the vehicle. Not only are we not the driver, we are sitting in the back.

Who is driving the vehicle? Our higher self is. This is why it feels as though we have no choice or control over our bodies, the vehicle.

In truth, however, we do have choice. If we work with our higher selves. First we must remember that our higher self is a part of us and we need to work as a team.

Through meditation and spiritual awareness we become the front passenger of our vehicle. Our higher self is still ultimately driving the car and overriding any decisions or desires we, as the passenger, might have, but when we are in the front seat, we are at least communicating with the driver about where we want to go.

Our higher self only wants to keep us on track with our purpose and lessons in this life. Therefore, if we communicate desires to our higher self, our higher self is often more than willing to assist us. However, if our higher self deems that the desire is not in keeping with our higher purpose, then it will override us.

If we do not meditate and focus on a spiritual path, we do not work in unison with our higher selves and we remain a back seat passenger who may shout out orders and desires, but is never heard or given much attention.

What we also learn by connecting with our higher selves through meditation is that we can learn our lessons in a positive way and can change basic patterns that were created before birth.

With this understanding also comes responsibility, for once you realize that you are the conscious creator of your existence in the body, then you can no longer blame anyone for how it works out.

You, in unison with your higher self, have the power to change your life and more importantly, to change the way you live and the way you create. The way to change this is by awareness first that you have that power and by moving within through meditation and a connection to your higher self.

The more we show our higher self that we are capable and responsible, the more our higher self will allow us to decide which route to take in our vehicle.

People often ask me why a child would choose to create a disease or death soon after being born. The answer is, to teach. Usually the child would be assisting the parent in learning about grief or loss. As spirits, we often come into bodies to assist others to learn something. It is the parent who is still in the body that suffers, not the child who has left, or perhaps in the case of disease, the child was merely choosing to experience physical suffering.

We all choose physical suffering at some time in our evolution but somehow we think that it isn't so bad when you are an adult. Actually, as a spirit choosing to experience something, it doesn't matter at what age the experience is undertaken. Often, if the spirit learns the lesson from the experience early on, then they will leave the body at a young age or sometimes incorporate another experience into the lifetime as well and stay longer.

The difficulty with choice which most people have is the question of murder. They cannot reconcile how anyone could possibly choose to be murdered. Especially to be murdered in some of the horrific ways that we regularly hear about on this brutal planet of ours.

The answer is of course, that we as human personalities are not choosing the experience of murder, but rather, we the spiritual selves, are, and usually before birth.

First of all, the experience of murder is a contract between two spiritual beings, each trying to help each other to evolve beyond the illusion of the planet and its suffering. The reason for choosing murder is usually to experience the emotion known as guilt. The experience is not so much a learning one for the victim, but rather for the murderer.

The murderer will always create a guilt from the experience, which is definitely one of the most difficult experiences on the planet, as it lingers for lifetimes and causes many other experiences as a result. For instance, in a future life one may experience unworthiness, fear, aloneness, as well as untold suffering that one creates to try to balance the guilt created by the murder.

For the person being murdered, they are usually just creating a way out of the body as they have completed with their lessons for that lifetime and are ready to leave.

We must find ways out of the body and we do so any way we can. However, the more connected you become to your higher self, the more you begin to create deaths which are easy and conscious. In other words, a lifting of your energy, rather than a struggle.

When death is understood as an illusion and an exiting, rather than a dissolving, there is no longer a struggle to stay in the body. When the struggle is not there, then leaving the body is easier.

We often create difficult deaths because we fear death so much and as such are learning about the fear we are creating in our minds, or because we are trying to hold onto the body so much, again because of fear.

Fear ultimately creates suffering of all kinds. We continually create our fears coming true until we finally learn that fear is our own creation. A creation of our ego because we no longer feel connected to our spiritual selves and therefore feel alone and insecure.

By the simple understanding that we are creators of our existence, we begin to take the power into our own hands. We work together with our higher selves and no longer exist as ignorant victims, but rather, as powerful and spiritual beings.

CHAPTER ELEVEN

Death

DEATH IS AN ILLUSION. WE do not truly die and dissolve into nothing. Nor do we maintain our physical forms and enter a paradise place in the clouds where we all sit around eating ice cream or playing golf throughout eternity, depending on your idea of what paradise is.

Throughout history religious leaders and philosophers have spent their lives preaching to us their ideologies about what happens after death.

During the dark ages, politicians and religious leaders began to focus more on the fear aspects of death rather than the heavenly ones. This enabled them to control people, as the concept of hell for eternity was an ingenious propaganda tool that put the fear of God into everyone.

Since the beginning, death has been a hotly debated subject, but one with little emphasis on truth. Politicians and religious leaders discussed and probably fantasized about what happened after their bodies stopped breathing.

If you look at the many religious teachings on our planet over the last six thousand years or so, most believed in some sort of after life, but exactly what that after life was is where disagreement and fantasy have flourished.

In my many studies of religious and philosophical beliefs from Christianity, Buddhism, Hindu, Muslim, Jainism, among others, I have noticed that all focussed on guesswork rather than actual experimentation, or they relied on statements believed to have been received from higher sources through mediums, oracles or chosen ones.

It has been my path in this life not to rely on others' words or philosophies but instead, to find out for myself. That is the difference between a belief and knowing. Belief is an idea which someone has taught to you and which you have adopted as your own. Knowing is a personal experience which you have encountered.

When you take someone else's word for something, you are giving your power away to them and also limiting yourself. Throughout history we have been a people who have followed blindly as a handful have attained bliss or enlightenment. Then we have blindly followed those who blindly followed the enlightened ones. We began to take those followers and enlightened ones words as the words of truth and never bothered to test those truths and find our own paths.

Often we have been taught by the followers that we were unworthy or unable to find such enlightenment ourselves and should be grateful to simply accept that those experiences happened and therefore follow the teachers words without bothering to find our own truth.

Whenever a being experiences something and then passes the wisdom onwards through words, it is guaranteed that those words will be distorted somewhat, or as often is the case, enhanced and embellished. Then that person passes on the words and again the meaning is even more distorted.

These are the teachings that we have blindly followed throughout history without questioning or searching for ourselves.

During my own spiritual path I have found two ways of answering the question of death. One is by journeying into the subconscious mind and remembering my deaths from past lives. The other is by having what is commonly called an out of body experience. Both can lead you to an understanding once and for all about the question of death.

Death, therefore, is not death at all, but birth. In some ancient cultures people used to weep at the birth of a child and celebrate a person's death. They understood that a birth meant that a spirit was entrapped yet again in a body for a lifetime and that death meant a freeing of one's spirit into a greater oneness.

It's interesting how modern cultures have switched it around and celebrate a birth and weep at a death.

By remembering our past lives using the technique of past life regression, we remove our fears of death and come to welcome it or at the least understand it as a changeover, a freedom, not a destruction.

I also feel it is important for us, as a culture, to witness death more often. It's common today for people to be taken to hospitals and to die alone. This creates a greater fearfulness in those left behind. A hundred years ago and beyond our loved ones died with us and us with them. This is an important part of life that we often miss.

Thirteen years ago I was with my niece when she died. I held her arm as her mother cradled her from behind. We sang her favorite songs to her as she slowly died. I felt that it was one of the most profoundly beautiful experiences of my life and certainly one that will linger with me forever.

I truly felt that her spirit was lifting from her body and freeing itself from a diseased physical form, which had been tortuous for her to live in. I also recognized that I was the only one present who truly felt joyous about the experience. To me it was a celebration, not of her life, but of her spiritual freedom.

Here was a spirit who would once again know complete unconditional love without egos and aloneness any longer. How could I be sad?

Those around me focussed on her body and found it very difficult to cope. A sadness did then arise in me, but it was not for her, it was for those who could not get beyond the fact that her body was dead. To them she was gone. Never to return. Lost.

To me she was found. She was out of the illusion and finally in truth. She had left her masks and the costume drama and could float in her pure energy self without any restrictions of a personality or a body.

Some time ago a person asked me if I agreed with the scientific community's desire to prolong life to infinity. She mentioned that she wanted to live forever and hoped that someday science would find a way, but recognized that it probably wouldn't be for hundreds of years.

I looked at her and felt my whole body sag as a wave of sadness swept through me.

"Why would anyone want to prolong life forever?" I said. "The very idea of wanting to stay in an illusion of heaviness, pain, ego and separateness for eternity is the saddest thing I have ever heard." "No", I said. "I would never want to stay in a body forever. The idea of staying for 60 or 80 years is hard enough, but eternity. Never!"

I understood, though, that her statement came from a place of fear and that made me feel even more sad. I realized at that moment how important it was to teach people the truth about death and why it should be embraced and welcomed, not feared.

To run from or avoid the most beautiful experience in existence is the greatest sadness in our world.

CHAPTER TWELVE

Karma

KARMA IS AN INTERESTING TOPIC that has been misrepresented over time. I recently walked into a new age store and noticed a sign above the cashier that said, "shoplifters will be subject to karma". I thought this was quite humorous although it did reflect what most people believe karma to be. Namely, what you have done to others will be done to you, or what you sow you will reap.

I find it has gotten a bad reputation that tends to cause fear in people and that is not, I believe, its purpose. Rather, karma is the natural law of cause and effect. When there is a cause or event created, then there will be an effect to that creation. Energy moves circularly and as such, must balance itself out. Karma itself is not negative or positive, it is simply energy, or intense emotion from an event that is trying to move in a circle and balance itself out.

When people think about karma they usually relate it to murder or negativity. If you murdered someone in a past life then that person will come back and murder you. Actually, that is not usually the case.

Karma can be positive as well. For example, love or kindness you have expressed will have an effect in the future, namely, something positive returning to you.

Karma does not balance itself in the exact manner of its original creation. It simply needs balancing in some way. What I try to do in regression therapy is heal karma in a positive way.

A young man came to me a number of years ago to try to help him uncover the reason for his desire to be Jewish. He was a young man of 28 with very blond hair and blue eyes and fair skin. Throughout his life he had a need to be accepted by Jewish people. His friends were Jewish and he longed to have a Bar mitzvah at the age of thirteen like other Jewish boys. The problem was, being so obviously Aryan in his looks, the Jewish community had difficulty accepting him as one of their own. He continuously struggled to be accepted by them and it was causing a great deal of torment in his life.

I decided to regress him into the cause of his problem. He found himself in Nazi Germany in World War II. He was a Nazi himself and was sitting at a table signing death warrants for Jewish people. At that time he had no remorse. He felt he was simply doing his job and somehow in his mind he justified it as necessary for his race's own survival. He then moved forward in time to a courtroom after the war had ended. He was being judged for war crimes and began to realize the extent of his mistakes. He was imprisoned and spent the next few years in torment over what he had done. He then hanged himself out of guilt.

After the regression he realized how he had been feeling guilty his whole life but didn't know for what. Obviously, he wanted desperately to be forgiven and accepted by the Jewish people that he had so carelessly sent to death in his past life.

Now it would have been easy if he had been born Jewish, but then he would have automatically been accepted. So he chose an obviously Aryan looking body so as to make acceptance and forgiveness difficult, as he carried a heavy guilt. He needed to prove his love to the Jewish people in order to balance out the past.

It was not necessary for the people that he had sent to death to come and kill him to balance the karma. In fact, the path he had chosen to balance the karma was quite positive.

Often we will spend many lives simply balancing out emotions and experiences created in a previous life.

For instance, if you have been an abuser of some kind then you will balance that experience by choosing a lifetime of abuse. Then the experience is complete and you have grown by learning both sides.

It has also been my experience that when you leave a past life, very rarely do you seek revenge. Instead, you seek balance.

For instance, on the other side of the Jewish/Nazi experience, I have regressed people who were murdered in death camps in World War II. To my initial surprise, none of them carried forward any anger towards the Nazi's themselves or any need for revenge.

When I asked them why during the regression, the usual reply was, "because they had chosen that experience and anger was not the experience, but rather, suffering was, as well as bonding and love with their fellow sufferers."

What is carried forward to be healed from past lives are unexpressed emotions. What may seem to us as a natural case for revenge is not always so.

I regressed a man to a life in the Holocaust. He was Jewish and was in a room with many other people. The room was being filled with gas and the people were dying. The man held his mouth to the crack in the door to try to absorb some pure air. Eventually, he died, as the others did, but during the process of death his experience was as follows.

He told me that he was experiencing a very heavy feeling on his chest and body and that he couldn't see anything, but he could smell gas. I asked him if he would like to move forward and through the death experience and he answered, "No". He said that he wanted to linger in this experience. That he felt it was important for him to remember the smell very clearly. He could not as yet explain to me what the heaviness on his body was or the fact that he could no longer see anything. I then asked him if he felt any emotions that he wanted to express. He said "No" again and that it was simply important for him to experience this lingering death.

After a brief while, I decided to ask him to move through his death and lift from the body. He did so and felt as though he was floating above his body from a great distance. He then told me that he left his body in a pile of other bodies, his being in the middle somewhere.

This explained why he had such a heavy feeling on top of him and why he could not see. I then asked him if he had any unresolved feelings towards the people that had murdered him and again he replied "No".

When asked the purpose of choosing such a death, he replied that it was important for his growth to understand how different cultures judge each other and torture each other in the name of their religions or beliefs. He said that rather than create an anger for him to balance in a future life, it created a greater empathy for all people on the planet, no matter what race, religion, or sex. He also said that he had learned about brotherhood and love with the other Jews he was with.

This man came to me because of a deep need to help people on the planet find peace and to better understand his path in this life. He is currently a ember of a world-wide peace organization.

On the other hand, sometimes a karmic circle will continue over many lives, but this is not usually the norm.

In order for a karmic pattern or circle to end, one person must be willing to heal the pattern and step out of the circle. Unfortunately, ego is involved and this often creates situations where neither is willing to express themselves honestly and emotions stay suppressed for lifetimes. All that is needed is for people to be honest and expressive in the moment and then energy is completed and nothing is carried forward to be healed.

Another often misunderstood reflection of karma is judgement. We see judgement everywhere in our lives and yet people continually deny that they are judgmental. It is interesting to see how often people judge each other and their habits only to discover that they had once done the same thing.

I had a female client come to me that could not tolerate her father's alcoholism and judged him heavily for it. When she went into her previous lives she experienced being alcoholic herself as well as abusive. It helped her to see more clearly her father's experience and to create empathy. She also realized that she was balancing her alcoholism from the past by seeing it from another perspective.

When you cause a negative or hurtful event in a previous lifetime it doesn't mean that the same event will happen to you, rather it does mean that the event will need to be balanced. However, sometimes, because we don't know any better, we will continue creating negative situations over and over with the same people and this creates what I call a "Karmic Merry-Go-Round".

When your spirit has chosen to balance a karma in a lifetime it does not necessarily choose how to balance it. Once in the body you take on ego and personality and, therefore, have conscious choice over how to balance the karma. This is how people can often get stuck on the Karmic Merry-Go-Round. They repeat the usually negative pattern the same as before without actually ending the pattern.

For instance, Sheila was a woman in her late thirties who had a bad experience with her sister, Beth, and she felt extremely angry and unable to forgive her sister. It had so disrupted her life that she felt an inability to trust others. Beth, had betrayed her years earlier by sleeping with her husband, who then left Sheila and ran off with Beth.

I regressed Sheila into a lifetime that she may have experienced with her sister Beth. She arrived in Bavaria as a young girl of seven who was playing with a neighbor of the same age. They were playing with dolls and when Sheila as the young girl was called in to the house by her mother, the young neighbor stole her doll and later lied about it. This caused a rift between the young girls that extended through their lifetime in Bavaria, as neither expressed their true emotions and healed.

In itself, that lifetime didn't seem to me to be enough cause for the anger and betrayal happening in the present life, so I asked Sheila if there was another lifetime she experienced with her sister Beth. She said there was.

She then found herself as a young man of twenty-two named Petra in Russia working as a stable hand on a grand estate. Petra was very poor and was jealous of the people who owned the estate and lived in such grandeur. As Petra looked around he noticed the young son who lived at the estate. The son came towards him in his shiny new embroidered silk coat and beautifully tailored clothes. He ordered Petra to ready his favorite horse for him. When Petra brought the horse the young man began to yell at him for failing to put the special new saddle on the horse. Later that night, Petra stole the young man's favorite horse as well as some gold goblets from the house and rode off.

As Sheila explored two more lifetimes the pattern became very clear. What began as one girl steeling a little doll from another little girl had escalated over many lives into steeling horses and eventually, husbands. I realized that Sheila needed to break free from the merry-go-round once and for all and balance the karma so she could move on with her evolution. In realizing the pattern, Sheila, during the regression, was able to forgive her sister Beth for the past as well as ask forgiveness herself from Beth's higher self to balance the karma.

Remarkably, a few months later, Sheila wrote to me and expressed how her sister Beth had telephoned her and said that her husband had left. She wanted to reconcile with Sheila and heal the wounds.

Interestingly, this is quite common. When one person heals or releases a past karmic link, the other person in the present also releases it, without even knowing why.

A man named Steve came to me for assistance with his friend. He told me that he had not spoken to his friend for a few months and there had always been a strange tension between them.

I regressed him into the cause of his difficult relationship with his friend. Steve found himself caught in a battle in the Civil War with his cousin fighting for the north and he for the south. During a battle he came upon a man who told him his cousin was nearby and wished to meet. He went to the rendezvous spot only to be ambushed and later imprisoned. While in prison, he wrote to the family and told them of his cousin's betrayal, whereby the family disowned the cousin and caused a breakage of communication between both sides of the family.

Naturally, upon remembering this, Steve released a deep feeling of betrayal and anger that had dogged him throughout his life. Then the negative energy between Steve and his friend was eliminated as Steve balanced the karma.

Another side of karma is creating and balancing positive experiences.

Linda had a past life as a wealthy socialite in pre-revolutionary France. She saw much poverty and illness around her and felt the need to help. She gave most of her money away to help the needy and began work as a midwife to poor women in need. The karma's effect in her next life was that of being greatly honored and loved by the people. Her next life was male and the people rallied around him as he lived a life as a dearly loved musician.

In the above experiences there had been an initial cause and then an effect to that cause in a future life. It is for you to choose whether that effect is to be negative or positive by being careful not to put out negative creations which will need to be balanced at a future time. The natural law says that it simply must be balanced to move on to the next lesson.

I had a friend who had a terrible time driving. He was often getting cut off by people and yelled at by them. In an experience looking through his past lives he came upon one where he had ridden chariots in Italy with great fierceness. He regularly ran people out of the way without the least concern for their safety.

Now when he drives he notices that people don't cut him off anymore because he asked for forgiveness in the regression to those whom he had injured.

Moving through our past lives gives us the opportunity to balance our karma more rapidly. To balance them we need to heal and complete the circle. This is done in the Astral or Bardo state where we call the energy of those with whom the karma took place and heal it by communicating and releasing the old energy. I will describe this in greater detail in a later chapter. Karma also doesn't necessarily have its balance in the next life. It is your choice as a spirit before coming into the body which karma you wish to balance in your next life. Often, in one life you may choose to balance many karmas.

The purpose of karma is to learn. If we only experience one side of things without experiencing the effect then we have not truly understood the lesson. All facets of life need to be tasted to truly find love and to evolve. To experience love, its opposite needs to be understood and experienced.

One thing I have certainly learned from karma is never to judge another's experience, for you either have been as they are or you will be.

We would all like to believe that in our past lives we were all wonderful, chivalrous, giving people. Unfortunately, that is not the case. We must experience both sides to balance and evolve with true understanding of the human experience. That means that we have been the bad guy as well as the good guy. The murderer and the victim.

This is not to say that it's alright to go out and murder people, but it must be understood that if someone murders, that person will have to balance it. It is not necessary or wise for us to be judgmental about another's experience, but rather to teach about the natural laws of cause and effect. Instilling fear in people will never teach them to stop hurting others, but teaching them about reincarnation and how they will have to balance what they are doing will teach people that they must have care with what they create. For in fact, if they harm another they are also harming themselves.

CHAPTER THIRTEEN

Soul Levels

THERE ARE MANY SOUL LEVELS that we move through in the cycle of death and rebirth in the human body. It is through these levels that we evolve and mature into wise, spiritual beings. It's like school. There is no set number of lives that we come here to live, we simply continue the circle of death and rebirth until we finally open our hearts and find only love. Not just for others, but ourselves and every part of existence. This is enlightenment.

We may experience ten or a hundred lives within each soul level, as there are many experiences to undergo and learn from in each level. It is up to us how quickly we grow.

In the following pages are the various stages of growth or evolvement that we go through in the human cycle.

You may notice that friends or relatives fit in to certain levels. In fact, we all fit in to one of them. It can be helpful in understanding our family when we can recognize what stage of growth they're at. Not to judge them, however, but to become more patient and accepting of them.

You wouldn't expect a child in kindergarten to act like a college graduate now would you?

So understanding where our friends and relatives are in their evolutionary path can help us to be more understanding and to let them be where they are without expecting them to be where we are.

INFANT SOUL

THE FIRST SOUL LEVEL IS commonly called the "Infant Soul". This level is experiencing their first incarnations in the human form. It is very awkward and uncomfortable and they often find it difficult simply getting through the day. They most often want to be alone as they find it difficult to socialize. Rather, this level is getting used to being in a body.

Most people in the Infant Soul level have no interest in bettering their lives by reading or education, they are simply existing and getting used to physicality. They will often create a very basic job with little mental stimulation and few social activities. Outside of their job they will usually focus most of their attention on food and basic comforts. They tend to lead quite isolated and quiet lives. The issues focussed upon are survival and little else. Just getting through the day is enough.

Towards the end of the Infant Soul level, they become more social and comfortable in their bodies and find themselves more interested in their outside world. Then they move into the next level, which is Baby Soul.

It's difficult getting used to all the complexities of a body and an ego and it takes many lives to get really comfortable.

BABY SOUL

THE NEXT SOUL LEVEL IS the "Baby Soul". This level is becoming much more socially adept and usually finds themselves very attracted to groups and organizations, clubs, etc. This is the level most associated with religion as they are very much seeking leadership but are not yet able to lead themselves. They are followers who tend to give their power away to others.

The Baby Soul begins to learn more about the world and starts educating him/herself. This level of soul is also very much focussed on procreation, which is why we call them "baby" souls. Naturally, this works very well in accordance with religion as religion promotes procreation heavily.

Sexuality is usually restricted to procreation purposes, however, not pleasure, although towards the end of the soul level they begin experimenting with sex a little more.

Sex is feared and often condemned because of the overwhelming power it has. The Baby Soul is also learning about control and fears anything that may cause it to lose control.

So the Baby Soul is happily evolving. They have gone from wanting to be alone to finding it difficult to be alone and always seek the company of others, whether in public places or by joining groups and organizations.

Socializing and creating babies as well as learning about concepts such as religion and a greater power is of prime importance.

They tend to place people on pedestals and are easily swayed into worshipping or becoming involved in organizations that use them.

They also often find themselves being victimized by others as they do not believe that they themselves have any power, so they willingly place their power in other people's hands and ask others to lead them.

By doing this they are hoping that others will fix their lives for them and are never willing to take responsibility for their own lives. They are always quick to blame someone else: governments, organizations, god, etc., when something doesn't work out in their life.

Baby Souls need to worship deities as they find it difficult to believe that they could have any power within themselves and are in awe of people that seem somehow close to a God, as they feel very separate and alone at this stage in their evolution.

Unfortunately, by worshipping, they are not recognizing the loving light within themselves and are distancing themselves even more from the spiritual energy within them.

As they evolve, they begin to absorb more knowledge and start to desire more, especially sex.

Because of their involvement with organizations that teach sexuality for procreation only, this often leads to repressed sexuality which turns to distorted sexual desires and habits as well as sexual crimes.

Then, on top of that, guilt and judgement are tossed in to make it more interesting and a vicious circle has begun.

It is most often in the baby soul stages that karma begins. As an infant soul we don't usually rack up any unresolved issues, but once sex and guilt comes into it, it's a whole new ball game.

YOUNG SOUL

THE THIRD LEVEL OF SOUL is the "Young Soul". This level is best described as the go-getter. They've experienced being led, are comfortable socially and with their bodies, and now are beginning to desire more, both sexually and materially. No longer are they satisfied with procreating and leading a simple religious life.

Now they look around and realize that something is not balanced. Some people have much more than others do and why should they miss out. So begins the quest for materiality and sensual satisfaction as well as ego gratification.

The young soul tends to have an abundance of energy. They often bounce out of bed at amazingly early hours and rush through their day seeking material goods and trying to satisfy their ever-hungry ego. They often have little patience and tend to suffer stressful illnesses as they have not yet learned to deal with the emotional self.

This level of soul focuses primarily through logic and intellect/ego. They avidly pursue education and knowledge, but only the type of knowledge that satisfies the intellect.

Often the Young Soul will pursue many educational degrees in order to become superior. This is the level of soul where competition is at its highest.

It was a Young Soul that created the saying, "The One Who Dies With The Most Toys Wins."

This soul is also very obsessed with showing off and seeking approval in the world. So they will continually seek out others to validate how great they are or to show off their toys and degrees.

This soul level likes to place all of their awards and accomplishments out for everyone to see. The degrees will be on the wall and the initials of the degree will be placed at the beginning or end of the name.

Sexuality as well will now become of primary importance and the young soul wants to experiment and taste all forms of it. They often become obsessed by it as well as other hedonistic pleasures until they are ready to evolve beyond it all.

The young soul is also sometimes called the "fun soul", as they have an abundance of dynamic energy around them. During the first two levels, their energy was growing steadily but had not as yet become very bright.

Now the energy is more expansive and directed outwardly into the world for others to see.

This soul will usually seek out fame and fortune in avenues such as stardom or political life where they have a good chance of being seen.

People are often very attracted to the young soul because they are so vivacious and exciting, but their pursuits are focussed on the material and the ego.

They are continually obsessed with their looks and want the adoration of others. A young soul will always ask, "How do I look?" or will discuss how much money they have or they will brag about their sexual escapades or intellectual achievements.

The reason is that it is not enough for the young soul to experience the pleasures of the body and ego, they must be honored for their achievements as well.

I have seen the subtleties of how the young soul seeks validation and it can be quite fascinating. Especially when it comes from the intellectual community. The intellectual mind/ego is continually trying to convince itself of its wisdom, and yet shows its insecurity by showing off its knowledge.

This is common in the world of universities and the so-called 'knowledgeable' set.

I recently went to a gathering where the room was filled with professors and the like who were continually trying to out-do each other with their expertise about various subjects. It fascinated me to watch them try to impress each other. Young souls at their best.

Although they try to prove how wise they are, they are doing it by simply parroting words and knowledge that they have accumulated from various books they have read.

Young souls will spend many years accumulating useless knowledge in order to convince themselves of their wisdom. The difference is that the wisdom they believe they have is actually just accumulated knowledge, which had been thought up by someone else or had been experienced by someone else.

For instance, during this gathering, a number of professors were discussing Aristotle and Buddha. They had all accumulated much knowledge, but neither had ever experienced anything of their own. They had never experienced what Buddha had and so could only discuss it.

This is the difference between knowledge and wisdom. Knowledge is someone else's experience, which you are learning about. Wisdom is your own experience.

That is also the basic difference between a young soul and an old soul. A young soul accumulates knowledge whereas an old soul must find their own wisdom by experiencing, rather than by just reading about how others did things or how others found enlightenment.

Now because the Young Soul has so much to experience and learn about, the majority of their evolutionary lives will usually be spent in this level.

They will start off learning all about their sexual desires through numerous lives spent exploring the many facets of sexuality. Then they will move on to lives of experiencing wealth, fame and power.

Eventually they will come to the intellectual pursuits and spend a number of lives exploring the capacities of their brain.

This is also when ego is at a peak. Spirituality is not felt, nor desired. The ego has you convinced the 'self' is mind and personality and that you are an 'individual'.

Because of this, the fun is over and the suffering is about to begin.

OLD SOUL

THE NEXT LEVEL OF SOUL is the "Old Soul". Old is right. By now the spirit has been in many bodies, maybe hundreds, and has experienced an awful lot of life. There can often be a sense of tiredness even in childhood.

This soul starts to question what the point is of the whole life thing anyway. I often call this level of soul the "tormented soul", for it is definitely the most difficult.

In the beginning of this level, the old soul tends to seek fulfillment from things that feel comfortable or familiar, which usually means by doing things that they have already done in previous lives.

For instance, they will dabble again in religion or the pursuit of materiality. The difference now is that none of the experiences of the younger soul levels will satisfy them any longer and the old soul becomes frustrated and often depressed.

Now because they have experienced so many lives in the past they will have an affinity and natural ability to create many things in their life, and often will jump from career to career in the search for something that fulfills. Unfortunately, nothing really does and the old soul keeps searching.

Eventually, this level begins to seek something else besides knowledge and begins the most profound quest of the inner self.

There is a gnawing feeling that there has to be something else to life than sex, money and knowledge.

Many old souls will spend much of their life doing what they have done in previous lives because it is easy for them. But soon boredom sets in.

An old soul will often change jobs not because of an inability to perform, but rather because the job is unfulfilling.

What begins to awaken is a deep hunger, almost an ache. This ache cannot be filled with worldly things but often the Old Soul will try. They try to purchase material things in the hope that they will fill the ache, but nothing seems to work. They will then usually try to create a greater activity in their life in order to avoid the constant empty feeling inside until finally they have to look deeper within for the reason for the emptiness.

Finally, the Old Soul begins the search for wisdom, not knowledge. Knowledge is someone else's experience, wisdom is your own. Wisdom comes from the inner self, whereas knowledge comes from the intellect.

The Old Soul begins to seek teachers rather than leaders, as they become unwilling to give their power away.

During this period of evolution, the soul also experiences the awakening of the deeper emotional self. Often they undergo profound emotional crises in order to better access their heart and inner self.

The Old Soul eventually begins to heal the pain of separateness and once again begin the path home to spirituality.

It is my opinion that the Old Soul level is the most difficult. It is at this time that the conflict awakens between the heart and ego and when the struggle to fulfill the emptiness inside is most profound.

The Old Soul is constantly seeking oneness and love while the world around is showing them separateness and fear. The challenge to the Old Soul is to be in the world and to be a loving spirit at the same time.

As this can be very difficult at times, it is quite common for an old soul to move through at least one life feeling lost and alone. They will often turn to numbing themselves because they are unable to deal with the pain of emptiness and lack of self worth that they feel. This is the level where addictive behavior is very common as well as madness, as the mind can often be very tormenting.

On the one hand, the mind is seeking fulfillment of the senses and the intellect, but the emotional self is seeking something greater. Often the person doesn't know exactly what they are seeking, they only know that there must be more to life than what they have experienced. This is where frustration, depression and sometimes madness can come in.

It is a part of the evolutionary path that all old souls must move through and thankfully, it is usually for only one life. If you know someone who is experiencing such a sense of being lost, it's important to have compassion rather than judgement for them. They are indeed moving through the greatest struggle in their evolutionary path. The struggle to find who they are and why they exist?

Eventually, the Old Soul will turn inwards and begin a path to understanding and finding self. This path may take many lives as the mind/ego will continually interfere and create postponements.

These postponements come in the form of relationships, desires, illnesses and various other distractions.

At some point the Old Soul also detaches from the chaos of the world as well as their attachment to things. They will move through regular cleansings in their lives, including cleansing their surroundings and ridding themselves of belongings, as well as cleansings of the body.

This is not to say an old soul must rid themselves of all belongings, but as a natural occurrence, the old soul simply finds that they are no longer attached to material things. They don't always get rid of them all, but if they were to disappear from their lives, they wouldn't be concerned.

People often try to become spiritual by ridding themselves of materiality and by abstaining from sex. It is important to realize that the spiritual journey can't be forced, it must evolve on its own.

You cannot push things from your life without having the desire return again and again. When you evolve, then naturally, you will lose the attachment to material things and you will eventually lose the desire for sex.

The problem that arises with people is that they try to abstain from desires and sex first and then the desires become a constant focus in their minds as does sex. They believe that to become spiritual they must abstain.

In truth, spirituality must come first and then desire leaves of its own accord.

If you try to suppress desire, it will become distorted. You must evolve beyond the desire.

If the desire is still there, it must be experienced until the desire holds no power any more. As a young soul there will be many desires and trying to suppress them will create a distorted mind and often a violent person.

I remember hearing many years ago an interesting statement by a spiritual teacher in India. He had no religious attachments whatsoever, he was simply an ancient soul teaching the way to enlightenment.

He was speaking about desires and in particular, sexual desires. His focus was on the habits of monks within particular Indian religions, although other religions certainly have the same patterns. He mentioned how the habit of religions was to put monks in a far away place where they could meditate and experience their spirituality. It was interesting to him that women were not allowed in these places. It was also said that these monks were very pure and had no sexual desires.

The teacher was quick to point out that when you run away to a mountain top retreat and take the desire away from one's daily contact, it is easy to pretend that the desire has indeed, been transcended. But was it really? How could you tell if the desire was really transcended if you never saw a member of the opposite sex?

The teacher thought it would be interesting to parade a beautiful naked woman in front of the pure monks to see who really had transcended desire and who had simply repressed it.

This brings us to an interesting point about spirituality. We must test our spirituality in the world. By hiding in a retreat it is very easy to be spiritual, but what about when we're in rush hour traffic in Los Angeles, or standing in a long queue when we have to go to the bathroom and the person in front of us smells of urine and is ranting about the alien spaceship that carried them off last night and took out their innards to have for dinner.

It is in daily living that we must test our spirituality, not by hiding away in monasteries or retreats. It's too easy there. One never truly knows if they are living a spiritual life or if they are avoiding life.

The process of enlightenment is a long one and will not be found in a few lives. All the experiences of aloneness, pain, and suffering will be experienced before one remembers who they are and that they are indeed, loving spiritual energy, deep inside.

As one moves towards enlightenment one becomes more humble and peaceful, one no longer creates roller coaster rides of the emotions and becomes more at peace with a gentle life as well as a quiet life.

We will often long for silence and nature and will have a greater respect for our bodies and will honor them by feeding them healthy food, rather than chemicals and abusive substances.

TRANSCENDENTAL SOUL

THERE IS ONE MORE LEVEL of soul I wish to mention and that is the "Transcendental Soul". This soul is simply a teacher. This spirit has remembered that they are light and one with all that is and decided to return to the human form to teach others.

Often these teachers become great master teachers such as Lao Tzu, Buddha, Jesus and Krishna. However, often they remain unknown to the massive public but bring light and peaceful understanding to many without asking for recognition and praise.

They do not brag about their spirituality, they simply teach and share it with others. They do not push their teachings upon others, but offer it with love. If others do not accept it, they are not bothered, nor are they empowered if people do accept it. It doesn't really matter to them if people embrace the teachings or not, they simply offer it to those who are willing to look within and find themselves.

The Transcendental Soul does not long to create followers or to be worshipped. They will actually push people away before they will encourage people to follow them. They teach empowerment not enslavement. They teach people to find their own truth, not to follow another's. They offer tools to help us find our truth, but encourage us to find it ourselves.

As in the master Buddha, he pointed a finger to the moon and asked not to look at his finger, but to look where he was pointing. In other words, don't focus on him, the teacher, focus on the teachings.

CHAPTER FOURTEEN

Out Of Body Journeys

IN THE LATE 1970's MY father died and I had clearly felt his presence around me for a period of three months. He would do various things that would startle me and cause me to know without a shadow of doubt that it was indeed, him.

I discussed the experiences with my doctor at the time and she recommended a book which had just come out called "On Death and Dying" by Elizabeth Kubler-Ross. At the time this book was a breakthrough in the question of life after death. Dr. Kubler-Ross had done extensive studies with patients who had experienced near death or had in fact been pronounced clinically dead and had returned to life. These people spoke about their experiences after their deaths. The experiences they spoke of were of floating above the body and being perfectly coherent as they watched their body beneath them.

The book fascinated me at the time as I had truly felt my father's spirit with me, but still something was missing. It was someone else's experience that I was reading about and not my own, so how could I truly understand or embrace it completely?

A part of me wanted to believe in an after life, as I wanted to believe that my father was really around me, but the other part felt the need to find out for myself rather than rely on someone else's research or experience or the Christian teachings I had been brought up with, which I felt no longer had anything to offer me.

I became hungry to get out of my body myself and began to read the few books I could find on the subject at the time.

It took me a few years, but one day as I was meditating on my couch without any expectations or desires, I felt a pulling sensation on the top left side of my head and shoulder. I watched the experience with a sense of detachment and allowed myself to flow with it until I felt myself pulled halfway out of my body by about two and one half feet.

Over the next year I began to have complete out of body experiences and found myself floating above my body and near to the ceiling and looking down to see my body still sitting on the couch.

When I first experienced completely leaving the body and then coming back into it, something had profoundly changed in me.

Upon lifting I felt myself much larger and more expansive than when I was in the body. I also felt an immense sense of peace and love. Gone was the busy mind chatter and the desires as I floated without an awareness of time or even of breathing.

I have no idea how long a time I floated out of the body as it seemed as though time was transcended. There were no real thoughts either, rather more of a knowingness and wholeness, feelings rather than intellectualizations.

When I came back into the body, I experienced a great heavy and cumbersome feeling. It wasn't very pleasant and I immediately wanted to get out again.

As I sat there and reconnected with my body, which was very stiff for a few minutes, I realized something profound. I welcomed death. The fear had completely gone and I actually looked forward to leaving completely and not returning.

I knew that I would not consider destroying my body to attain death, but that I could look forward to the lifting out and moving into that peace.

When I walked around I felt awkward. It seemed such a burden and almost ridiculously funny to move within this almost foreign costume again. It was then that I began to call my body, "my costume" or "armor", as it seemed just that.

I had experienced my true self, spiritual energy, for the first time and I no longer felt that I was the body or the personality. This event truly set me on a spiritual path. Everything and everyone around me seemed different.

I noticed when I went to work how everyone was so caught up in their personalities and their bodies and it tormented them endlessly.

I felt a new-found freedom and a sense of sadness for those around me. It was as though I began to see life from a distance rather than being caught up in the drama.

The more I experienced out of body journeying, the more at peace I became. I knew completely and without a doubt that I was not a personality or a body, but a spirit and this knowing brought a sense of relief and joy such as I had never experienced and which is difficult to put into words.

Life became more fun for me because I no longer felt trapped. Although whilst in the body I never realized that I felt trapped, as soon as I lifted from it and returned I realized that I had felt stuck or trapped and had longed for the freedom and lightness of being that I was now experiencing.

An out of body experience is not as difficult as it may seem either. Throughout time people have been experiencing them and often as children we experience them and then forget how to as we grow.

In my studies of out of body experiences, I have come across many people who have stated that they often find themselves having an out of body experience during the night.

One such subject, Sheila, mentioned that she had been asleep and had been slowly awakened by a sense of needing to go to the bathroom. She felt herself rise from bed and move towards the bathroom. When she tried to sit on the toilet she felt unusual, as though she could not get down far enough. When she focussed on looking down at herself she could not find her body, but since it was dark she didn't really question it. She then realized that she no longer felt as though she had to pee, so she returned to her bedroom where she received an incredible shock. She saw her body lying peacefully asleep in bed.

Stunned by her discovery, Sheila suddenly felt herself pulled rapidly back into her body. She sat up suddenly and felt her heart pounding in her chest and her whole body vibrating intensely with energy.

This is actually a common experience for many people. Because you are made of what scientists call "Quantum Energy", it is your energy that begins to separate from your body when you are very still for a period of time.

During sleep or in a meditation, your energy begins to expand from the confines of the physical body, as though the boundaries of the body no longer are able to contain the energy unless it continually moves. This stillness allows you to stretch your energy and to lift out.

Most people find it easiest to lift from the physical at about 3:00 am when they have been asleep and then gently awakened.

In one of my first experiences with out of body, I too was awakened by a gentle thud sound in the middle of the night. I awoke to find my whole body vibrating and buzzing with an electrical feeling. This is our true self, vibrating energy. When I awoke I thought that maybe the sound had been created from my cat and that I should go and check on him.

To my surprise instead of lifting my body out of bed, I began to feel my face being pulled out and soon I was sitting upwards in bed, but my body was not. I then lifted completely up and floated down the hall where I found my cat sound asleep on the couch. I then experienced what many do when having out of body experiences, I thought about my body back in bed. At that very moment I felt myself pulled swiftly back into my body. I opened my eyes and felt the same experience that Sheila had, a rush of energy and my heart pounding with excitement.

Most people who have out of body experiences, however, have them because of an injury or accident, or a near death experience. When the body experiences a sudden impact of say, a car accident, your energy can actually pop out of the body. The spirit then finds itself suddenly floating above the accident and watching the whole thing with a sense of confusion.

One of my earlier clients had told me about an experience she had when she had drowned and been brought back to life. She mentioned that after she had stopped struggling she began to feel quite euphoric. See saw beautiful colors all around her and felt peaceful and safe. Then she felt herself begin to float upwards. She looked down and soon saw her body floating face down in the water and felt no desire to re-enter it. After a few moments of watching this some people dragged her body out of the water and began to give her mouth to mouth resuscitation. During that time, she felt confused as she experienced a pulling sensation towards her body.

She told me then that she felt very reluctant to return to her body and wanted the people to stop trying to resuscitate her. Then she felt pain and a heaviness and realized that she was back in her body. When she regained consciousness she told me that she was angry and felt depressed. When I asked her why, she said because when she was floating above her body she felt so full of love and peace and since coming back she no longer was able to feel it.

I then encouraged her to learn to travel out of her body. It took her some time, approximately a year, but she eventually did and told me that she was so happy to be able to re-experience the freedom of her spirit. She also told me that she looked forward to leaving her body for good, but recognized that she had a purpose and would see it through and for the first time, actually loved her body.

The out of body experience is truly a wonderful way to feel your true self and to experience the joy and freedom of your spirit. People have asked me if it would not encourage suicide? I can honestly say that all of those people that I have talked to that have experienced an out of body have a greater reverence for life and for their body and would not harm it in any way.

I have noticed in working with people who have been through very traumatic issues in their lives such as sexual abuse or violence, that when one feels trapped then there is often a longing to get out and to think about suicide. However, when you experience an out of body journey, you no longer feel trapped and so it actually eliminates any desires for suicide.

When you know you can leave any time, you find that you can enjoy life and the body even more, because you do so with a sense of detachment. You begin to see life as a creation of experiences and lessons and not as a curse. No longer do you feel a victim but rather a powerful creator, and you no longer fear death.

During the out of body experience, one usually feels a tremendous love and peace and often a brightness of light. I have noticed that if people have a Christian background, this is often interpreted as been a deity who has come to guide them or lead the way. Rather, if one has a Buddhist or Taoist background, they usually feel that it is not a separate being that has come to them, but it is actually universal energy that they are rejoining with. A part of themselves that they have been separated from. This has also been my experience.

During my upbringing as a Catholic, I was taught to believe that when you die then all of your dead relatives and friends come to meet you and help you through the passage. This was something that I later wondered about and felt the need to research further.

In my questioning of many people who had experienced actual out of body experiences, I found that they all experienced the same thing, a brightness or light around them and a warm loving and peaceful feeling. None told me of any meetings with other spirits or relatives.

In later questioning people who had various religious beliefs, I found that those with Christian teachings believed that they met loved ones, but those of other backgrounds never had heard of such a thing. Naturally, this aroused my suspicions once again. Was more propaganda at work in the Christian teachings? It certainly seemed so, as no one I had spoken to who had left their body had ever experienced other beings coming to them, but neither did they feel an absence of them. They in fact felt very much a part of everyone and everything, no longer separate or in need to meet an old relative or loved one.

In discussing out of body experiences with people and having my own, I found myself limited in one area. All of us had come back and lived, so none of us could comment on what happened when we actually died or stayed dead. In other words what happened next? Did we continue to float over our bodies for eternity or move on to some other place? This was a question that no one could answer to my satisfaction without simply theorizing and bringing up old religious concepts. That may be fine for a follower, but I wanted to know, not believe. I knew that I could never be satisfied with some ancient teachings because how did they know? Besides their experience was not my own. This ultimately led me to past life regression.

I understood the teachings of reincarnation and had experienced a few past life regressions of my own but had not moved through any death experiences. I realized that it was through the memory of my past deaths that I would find the answers.

I began my research in two ways, my own experiences and by taking others through their past lives and their past deaths. The culmination of this twenty-five year experiment of over 2,000 people is this book.

CHAPTER FIFTEEN

The Bardo/Astral State

IN TAKING OTHER PEOPLE THROUGH their past lives and then their death experiences, I was fascinated by the fact that they would always tell me the same basic things. I developed a number of very simple questions to ask them about what they were experiencing, as I understood the necessity to never lead someone during a regression. One reason for that is that the person will usually become annoyed at you, because no one wants to be lead and, secondly, it only creates confusion in the person and then they stop communicating with you.

The easiest thing to do when regressing someone is to ask very basic questions, such as, "What are you experiencing?" or, "What are you feeling?" Little more was necessary to ask as the person was always willing to tell me what was happening to them.

In regressing over two thousand people through their past lives and deaths and regressing myself through approximately fifty, I found the similarities extraordinary.

When first feeling the death experience beginning, we feel a sensation of being pulled or lifted upwards. In some cases there is a reluctance to leave, depending on the situation the body is going through, but in general, there is a feeling of acceptance and calm.

We then feel ourselves lifting out of our bodies and are sometimes surprised that we feel no different, except any pain and struggle is suddenly gone. A sense of lightness and warmth comes over us similar to that experienced in an out of body journey. We then usually look back down and find our bodies which have become still.

The first sensations at that point are of tremendous freedom and expansion, as when you take off a shoe that has been too tight and hurting your feet. A feeling of relief flows through you and a wonderful sense of peace.

Next we become aware of a tremendous light around us and a warm loving feeling that surprisingly seems to come from not only around us but from inside us. As though our love has suddenly been freed and is expanding within us.

If we have a connection to family members or other loved ones left behind, it is common to stay around the body for a period of time, which can be anywhere from a few days to years.

We, as spirit energy, will float around and try to communicate with our loved ones to bring them comfort, but usually we give up after a while when we realize no one is paying attention or able to receive or sense us.

When I asked people how they felt about being dead during their regressions, some would laugh softly or purse their eyebrows as they replied, "but I'm not dead, I'm right here and I feel more alive than I ever did in the body."

People often expressed to me that they felt much larger than they had before and when I would ask if they felt any desire to return to the body they would quickly reply, "No way, this is too wonderful. I want to stay here forever."

Often the spirit then finds itself swirling and spinning or just enjoying the sensations of floating and of course, of love and peace. Sometimes they would express to me that no words could adequately convey the totality of oneness they were experiencing, nor how pure love really was.

It was incredible to me how people would regularly mention that the love they experienced in the body was so small or limited compared to the complete and unconditional love they were experiencing now.

It was during these realizations of my own and through my research of others' experiences that I realized how our expressions of love whilst in a body are often tainted by the mind and by the desire for control or need. It's as though love in the body is masked by the ego and not truly expressed or felt, whereas once you leave the body love becomes much more pure and whole.

When the spirit feels it is time to move onwards and no longer stay to comfort the relatives, it moves to the next level of the in between life state, which we call the Bardo (a Tibetan term for in between lives) or the Astral. This is the level that we have been unable to experience in a near death or out of body and can only be remembered during a past life regression.

When one moves through the death, one feels and senses a tremendous light around oneself and a loving sensation within. When one has completed with the body and relatives, then one is ready to rejoin or reconnect with the higher energy or higher self as it is often called.

The light that is around you is actually your higher energy, an energy that you split from when you came into the body and one that you will now rejoin with. This next stage of rejoining is a stage of incredible love and bliss.

The lighted energy actually permeates you and you again become one. A sense of greater expansiveness and wisdom is again re-experienced and an understanding of the universe and life itself.

It is at this stage that I would ask questions such as, "What is the meaning of life?" and "Why did you come into the body?"

I was thrilled to find that without fail, people responded with the same answers. They told me that the meaning of existence was to find love and to grow or expand. That they were a part of the universal energy but had chosen to separate to a degree long ago to undertake a new experience of understanding love.

They explained that as universal energy, or the God force, they had been an expression of pure love, but in order to fully understand that love, they chose to step outside of it and forget and then to undergo difficult lessons in order to re-experience love. Then they would truly know love.

Only through separating from love and looking at it through the guise of aloneness or fear would they then be able to truly understand what love was and then embrace it fully again. They needed to experience the opposite of love in order to know true love and the experiences of humanness, like suffering and judgements, were definitely the opposite of love.

It seemed to me almost the experience of a child needing to separate from parents to undergo lessons and experience separateness and then to grow to old age where there would, hopefully, be a greater wisdom.

Invariably, everyone would also state to me that they were not told or forced to come into a body but that they had, in fact, chosen to enter the cycle of death and rebirth.

During this state of awareness when we are rejoined with our higher selves, we realize that we are in fact, the creators of our bodies and our very existence. There is a realization that in this rejoining we have reconnected with our better half, so to speak.

I find it interesting that throughout our lives we find ourselves seeking a mate, which we often refer to as our better half. Rarely does that relationship, or any other, satisfy our deepest needs and longings. I firmly believe that the endless longing for another part of ourselves to make our lives whole is actually the search for our higher self which we separated from in the birth experience.

Once we reconnect with this higher self, we understand that we are, indeed, the creators of our existence and bodies, but also that we are not alone and never were. Unfortunately, when we are in the body we forget this and usually feel as though we are moving through our existence completely alone and often, misunderstood.

I think it is very important to teach our children and help ourselves to reconnect with this higher self while still in the body, so that we feel that connection to our higher spirit and never feel the aloneness that so often causes pain in our lives.

Rarely does a person go through life without feeling a deep aloneness at some time. This can often cause great despair and even thoughts of suicide. When you move through a past life regression and experience that unification with your higher self it is a tremendously joyful reunion and changes your life, because you know from that moment on that you are not alone and never will be. It also encourages people to continue to pursue a greater connection with their higher selves through meditation.

During the regression, whilst in between lives, the spirit finds itself moving into yet another layer in the Bardo state where they begin to look back and examine the past life they have just experienced. They look back to understand the lessons and experiences that were chosen prior to birth and to discover if all of the lessons were indeed learned in that life, or if they are going to carry something forward to be completed in a future life.

This is also where karma is actually decided upon. People often feel that karma is thrust upon them, but actually, it is also chosen.

Karma is the natural law of cause and effect. If there is a cause in a lifetime that has not balanced, then during this state of the Bardo you will decide what to carry forward to be balanced in a future life. All karma must be balanced at some point or another, but you choose which life to balance it in and how to balance it.

This level of the Bardo or Astral is also where one heals issues during a past life regression that were not dealt with in the past life and issues that may be carried forward which are effecting you in the present.

When looking back on your past life from this viewpoint, it is easier to understand the whole picture of the life and to find answers to the most profound questions, such as, "Why did you choose that particular life" and "What did you learn." This is where you would normally spend the most time in a regression releasing any pain and unhealed emotions from the past which will free your present life and help you to heal.

After the spirit moves through this phase of examination of the life, it is ready to move to an awareness of rest and peacefulness. It is important to note here that the examination of the past life does not include being judged in any form whatsoever.

So often in our religious teachings we have been taught that we will at some point after our death be judged by some panel or greater being who will decide if we've been naughty or nice. This simply does not happen. You look back to understand what you have learned and how much you have evolved, not to be judged.

On occasion one may sense the presence of a higher "guide" or helper spirit to assist you in understanding how you have grown, but this spirit is not there to judge you.

I have actually been quite fascinated to find that rather than being judged by other spirits, or deities, we tend to judge ourselves.

When we have experienced a life where we have been hurtful to others or even committed some heinous acts, we find it easy to judge ourselves during this examination of our past in the Bardo state.

The complete love and acceptance that we feel from the unification with our higher selves and sometimes the presence of an assistant spirit or guide, helps us to understand that all life experiences are simply to be understood as lessons and it doesn't help us to punish ourselves or others.

Although it is necessary to balance those deeds in order to heal and evolve, we are not punished or judged by any spiritual being. Rather we are helped to understand the pain and suffering caused by an absence of love and oneness and, therefore, encouraged to love more and to help others, rather than destroy them.

The rest period we move into next is just that, a time to rest in the wholeness of universal energy. During this phase there is an awareness of simply floating in love and silence. This period may last anywhere from about 40 days to 400 years. Time is actually no longer applicable once you have left the physical dimensions and entered the astral dimensions.

As has often been discussed by those who have experienced an out of body journey, once you leave the body you are also leaving linear time and moving into a state of now. This concept is completely foreign to our logical minds as we are firmly rooted in linear time. The only way I can help you to understand it is to encourage you to try an out of body journey, then you will understand the absence of time, maybe not logically, but intuitively.

I have also discussed the subject of time with many in the spiritual community who have had similar experiences to my own and they too find it difficult to put it into a logical perspective.

The idea often arises that everything is happening now because there is no linear time and therefore, lives do not necessarily happen in a linear pattern. I tend to disagree with this because of my experiences and research with regression.

People have argued with me that you should be able to have a lifetime say now, in the twentieth century, and then, arguably have your next one back in the dark ages.

I understand this concept but it doesn't quite work for me. Of all the regressions I have taken people through, they always remember them in a chronological manner. In other words, they move through their lives in a linear pattern and leave no space for themselves to suddenly jump back and experience a life a thousand years ago.

I also feel that this would make it difficult for the evolutionary growth pattern to work and for karma to work.

I do, however, agree that the experience of linear time is limited to the physical plane as I myself have experienced moving out of it during an out of body experience. However, I feel that as we have chosen to be a part of this experience of physical form, we have also chosen to be a part of the illusion of linear time.

Clearly, the body is an illusion as well and yet we accept that quite readily so why wouldn't we accept the illusion of time as well.

During my rigorous questioning of clients during the Bardo state they have repeatedly stated that universal energy or Light created the planet as a school of sorts to learn to understand love and to evolve to a heightened energy.

If we as spiritual energy accepted being a part of this illusion of physical form and separateness why wouldn't we also accept a linear procession of lifetimes in order to grow and find our truth.

It doesn't make sense to me to have lives scattered through time where we are bouncing from the dark ages to the future and back again. If there were a purpose to it, then I would give it further warrant, but as yet I have found none.

Through the examination of my own lives and others, each lifetime has immediately been followed by another where karma is usually carried forward and then, balanced. If we jump all over the place, that would make it impossible to balance lives.

Through the examination of our creation and the movement through reincarnation to ultimately find our truth, I find quite a logical understanding in the process of beginning, growth, and then completion. I see it as necessary in coming into such an illusion as bodies, egos and planets, that we would have to create something such as linear time in order to experience growth and evolution.

Yet, once beyond the circle of reincarnation, when we completely rejoin with universal energy through the process called enlightenment, then I feel the illusion of linear time would be completely transcended and nowness again a part of our understanding. But then, separateness is also transcended and all other illusions as well.

To put it plainly, we have chosen to be a part of this illusion called physical form and with it we take on the various illusions that go with it, including time, gravity, mind and ego.

As we move out of our blissful resting period as a spirit, we are ready to begin to choose our next lives. During a regression this is often a most fascinating exercise in remembering and understanding choice.

During a regression a client would often be surprised when they told me answers to such questions as, "Why are you coming back into a body", and "Which sex will you have".

In the beginning of my research with past life regression and reincarnation I was stunned by the answers I would hear during this phase of the Bardo state. Here, people would tell me that they were choosing everything, including their sex, their parents, their basic lessons to be learned in the coming life and very often, their death. They would also tell me of specific events they were choosing in order to learn from, including an illness, trauma, war or conflict of some sort or even an exciting or wonderful event.

It is in this stage that we create a basic blueprint for our next life in order to best learn the lessons we are choosing. Often we simply choose one lesson, for instance, anger or joy, creativity or ignorance, suffering or fear. We also choose what karma to bring forward to balance in this next life.

We may also linger in this state as we allow circumstances to create on the planet that best suits our choices. For instance, if we really want to be born into a certain family and have a certain mother that perhaps you want to balance something out with and learn from, it may be necessary to wait for her to grow up and marry before you come back as her child. Or, you may be choosing to experience a certain world event with others and therefore, have to wait until circumstances create for that world event.

During this creative process, it is also important to realize that other beings are also creating their next lives. This begins what we call mass consciousness creation.

When many beings long to create or learn from a certain experience, such as a war, then the output of their energy creates the experience so that they may all be a part of it.

During this time of choice we must remember that when another being is involved in our lessons, they have choice as well.

For instance, if you are choosing a certain woman to be your mother then she must be willing to accept you as her child otherwise she does not have free will and would merely be a victim, right? But how does she make that choice if she is already in the body and is going through life busily focussed on school and hasn't a clue that a spirit wants to come through her and be her child.

What happens in this case is that the mother's higher self which stays in the Astral dimension, will receive the desire from the spirit to be the child and the higher self will then make the decision.

A spirit can never force their will on another without their being a contract between the two higher selves, although rarely does one recognize this contract consciously because once you have come into the body you have disconnected once again from your higher self and have forgotten everything.

This is why most people go through their lives feeling and believing that they are victims and why it's so important to reconnect with your higher self so that you can consciously know what choices are being made and be a part of that creation, rather than a victim of it.

This leads me to the next phase of the Bardo state which is when your spirit moves closer towards the body and a new life again.

After you have chosen the basic blueprint of your life and there is acceptance from the higher self of the mother to receive you, then you move closer to the mother and also to the father. It is also a part of your experience to be around when you are conceived. You are a part of the creation, after all.

This is quite hilarious for people during a regression and sometimes people choose just to skip it as most find it hard to watch their parents making love. Nevertheless, you were there and it is a part of your memory, whether you want to remember it or not.

This next level of your spiritual path is quite important to your later experiences within the body as it is during this next nine month growth of your foetus that some emotional experiences may set up your future emotional well being.

During this phase you, as a spirit, hover around the left shoulder of your mother. You are a whole, circular lighted energy and you float alongside her throughout the pregnancy.

I find it interesting that throughout history people have stated that pregnant women glow. Well, no wonder, there is a glowing light hovering beside them.

What few people have realized during the term of pregnancy is that the spirit is outside the mother's body and not inside it.

This realization answers, once and for all, the question of the foetus being a separate being before birth and the question of ethics regarding the issue of abortion, as the spirit does not enter the body until just prior to birth.

This is, however, a very important period to the spirit. Throughout the pregnancy the parents and others are talking about the baby as though it cannot hear and they never realize that the spirit can not only hear everything that is being said around it, but it also sees everything and absorbs everything related to it.

So often I have worked with people who have had difficulty with self worth and happiness or acceptance through their lives and have had no real basis for that unworthiness. In taking them into regression and simply suggesting they go to the root of their unworthiness, invariably they would arrive at this stage where they were floating beside their current mother and listening to everything being said about them.

As is often the case with a new mother, worry and fear arises about her pregnancy and whether or not she can care for it properly or perhaps, whether she will be a good mother. Also there are often times where the mother is experiencing an argument with the father about the pregnancy or even someone else, such as her parents.

What has never been realized before, is that the spirit is right there watching and listening to all of this.

To understand it more I will give you the case of Melissa.

Melissa had come to me at the age of 43, feeling unworthy and unloved. She was never able to create a relationship or joy in life and she could never understand why.

When I asked her about her childhood and anything about her birth that she had been told, she said everything had been wonderful. Her parents both adored her since birth and throughout her life she had experienced a normal childhood. Never had her parents or anyone else ever been cruel or made her feel unloved.

During the regression she found herself floating beside her mother just after her mother had found out she was pregnant. She watched as her mother looked terrified as she talked to a girlfriend, stating that she didn't want the child. She said the baby would ruin everything and that she would have to quit university and live a life of poverty. Melissa continued watching as her soon to be mother paced the room and talked about finding a way to abort the foetus.

Later, as the pregnancy evolved, Melissa found herself watching a fight between her father and mother about money and how the child would limit their lives. She heard her father say how he had wanted to travel to India and discover himself and now he couldn't.

During the regression, Melissa experienced herself becoming more and more depressed and a feeling of despair settled into her. She almost decided to disconnect herself from the situation and find other parents, but realized that she had chosen them for a reason and she still wanted to complete her lessons with them as her parents.

As is often the case, once Melissa was born, her parents immense love for her overwhelmed them and they never questioned their decision to become parents. Then as Melissa grew, she experienced a normal, healthy loving childhood and never understood where this continual feeling of unworthiness came from.

In looking back, she was able to understand her parent's initial fears and realize that they did truly welcome her once she was born.

What we can learn from Melissa's experience is that the period of pregnancy needs to be looked on with a new awareness and care. The parents need to realize that the spirit is actually outside the mother and very much aware of everything being said and done.

During the course of the pregnancy, however, the spirit also decides to dip into the foetus on occasion just to get a feel for things and to get used to the tightness and heaviness once again in a gradual way rather than being thrust into the foetus.

Rarely does the spirit linger for long in the foetus, however, as they find it constricting and uncomfortable and there is nothing to be experienced there, whereas there is much to be experienced by watching the mother and father.

It is during this watching, as well, that sometimes a spirit will change its mind as it realizes the parents may not be what they want. It then decides to leave, wherein the foetus will usually miscarry, or sometimes be stillborn if it is far along in the pregnancy when the spirit leaves.

The spirit may leave for any number of reasons, but mostly because it realizes that the parents are not right for its purpose in the coming life.

The spirit may be choosing a life of conflict and find the parents too nice or it may be choosing a life of great expression and finds the parents too stifling. In other words, there can be so many reasons for a spirit choosing to leave.

In the case of Moira, she was four months pregnant when she miscarried. As she was devastated, I encouraged her to connect with her higher self through meditation. As she had been an adept meditator, it was quite easy for her and she realized that the spirit that had originally connected with her was in fact wanting to experience a war or conflict in its life. Moira, a reporter, had earlier decided that she was going to spend her life travelling to countries in conflict, but when she became pregnant, she changed her mind as she felt it would be no life for a child. The spirit had only chosen her as a mother because of her choice to be a correspondent in war torn countries and so left when she changed her mind.

Throughout my years of working with people, I have found it fascinating to learn why a spirit will leave before birth and sometimes right after birth. I earned that we must not judge others for decisions of abortion, as the spirit is the one choosing to stay or leave in agreement with the mother's higher self.

Sometimes a spirit will also leave just after birth, such as is the case with Sudden Infant Death Syndrome. This is also a similar experience wherein the spirit has changed its mind and decided not to stay with those parents.

On occasion, however, a spirit will also come into a body and stay for only a short time in order to help the parents learn a lesson. This is where a further understanding of the agreements between higher selves can be understood.

For instance, a woman's blueprint before she chooses life again is to experience grief. As she becomes a woman and longs to become pregnant her higher self begins to create the circumstance in order for her to learn her experience of grief and, therefore, her lesson in the life she has chosen. Her higher self would then invite a spirit that is coming close to choosing a life and a contract would be made for that spirit to assist in the woman's learning by entering the body for only a short time.

This spirit is offering itself for a short while to assist in a learning experience. This one being grief. Often a spirit will do this that has had previous experience with that very same woman and is usually a part of her soul family. That is the extended spiritual family for which she belongs and who reincarnate with each other over and over again in order to teach each other and help each other evolve.

As the spirit is preparing to enter a physical form again, it needs to prepare itself, which it does by dipping into the foetus on occasion and becoming connected with the parents.

I have taken people into regressions to remember their pre-birth experience. They would explain to me how warm and tight it felt when they would dip into the foetus and sometimes, how reluctant they were to actually enter a human form again. The spirit seems to go through a phase of hesitation at this time before committing to the body once again. They recognize that it is a part of their spiritual evolution to continue the process of physicality and that they have in fact agreed to do so, but there is still a hesitancy, mostly because they realize what they are disconnecting from.

Although there is often a sense of anticipation at a new growth experience there is also a reluctance to leave behind the love and sense of wholeness and oneness with all that is. During this period a spirit may change its mind simply because it suddenly decides that it wants to wait a while longer and linger in spirit and light a little more before undertaking ego and separateness again.

It seems to me to be quite a courageous jump for a spirit to make. To detach from complete love and acceptance in order to enter an illusion filled with suffering and ego oriented societies seems to me not only courageous but also a little nuts. Still, we recognize that it is all a part of understanding love and oneness and we ultimately know in our spiritual selves that we will again return to that oneness and when we finally complete the cycle, we will be wiser for it and will return to the fullness of universal light and energy forever.

CHAPTER SIXTEEN

Soul Levels Of The Bardo

To FURTHER THE UNDERSTANDING OF the Bardo or Astral state, I will explain in greater detail the seven levels that spirit energy moves through when they leave the physical body. These levels are layers within the dimensional realm of the Astral or Bardo. A dimension is a vibration of energy which is always around us but is separated by a thin veil-like energy field which makes it difficult for us with our human eyes to see through.

After much research I have named these levels to better explain them. Other philosophical or religious teachings may have other names for them but I have not come across them.

The first level is the Mind Astral level.

You have probably heard about the experience of astral travelling or astral projection. It seems to be a common occurrence and much has been written about it. Unfortunately it has not been explained fully and it has also been thrown together with Etheric out of body experiences. In actuality the two are quite different.

The experience of moving onto the Mind Astral level is one of projecting energy from the third eye or forehead area of the head. This creates the visual experience of being somewhere else or of seeing or sensing other places and people.

This is the most common occurrence that people have and is often misunderstood to be an actual out of body experience.

Often in my teachings people would say to me, "I think I had an out of body experience where I was travelling over Europe somewhere." My reply would be, "No, you were not."

How could I be so sure? Because a true out of body experience is never mistaken or questioned. When you are having an out of body or etheric projection, you know it, without a doubt. On the other hand, when you are having a mind astral projection, you aren't sure of what exactly is happening.

With a mind astral projection you are taking a small amount of energy out of your head and projecting it to a certain place on the planet. This creates a vision of that place, usually vague. You see people moving about and doing their daily routines and are often confused by what you are experiencing because at the same time you are still aware of being at home and lying in bed or wherever you are.

With a mind astral projection you are still connected to your present body and you are aware of it. You are not really disconnecting from your body and so your projection seems vague and when it is complete you are often unsure of what you experienced. You can still be completely aware of your present body and its aches and pains or discomforts and so the vision you are seeing never really becomes lifelike. It is hazy and is often confused with having a good imagination. It is not, however, your imagination, it is an astral projection.

The second level of the Bardo state is the Etheric level. This is where one has an out of body experience or a near death experience.

Contrary to an astral projection where you are taking out a small amount of your energy from your head, an etheric projection or near death experience is the taking of most of your spiritual energy out of the body, leaving only enough to sustain the body's vital functions.

When you have an etheric projection you feel as though you are completely lifting out of the body, there is no question about it. You will usually find yourself floating above your body and looking down at it. This often creates unusual feelings in people because as they are floating they still feel as though they have their bodies with them.

The reason for this is that when you take your etheric energy out of the body it remains in the form of your physical body for some time. Eventually if you stay out long enough, which most people don't, your energy begins to lose its physical shape and become a more rounded form of energy.

People will often first experience a true etheric projection in the middle of the night when they get up to go to the bathroom. They arrive at the bathroom and find they have no body. Then when they return to their bedroom, they see their body still lying in bed, sound asleep.

The reason for this is that it takes a deep relaxed state to occur within the physical body before your energy will be able to release itself. Your body needs to be completely still for at least one half of an hour, and I mean completely still. Then your energy begins to loosen itself from the physical form.

This process happens to a great deal of people during their sleep but they are unaware of it. The only signs that it has happened if you don't remember it is that you have had the sensation of flying when you awaken the next day or you awaken and find yourself ravenously hungry.

People will usually confuse an out of body experience in their sleep with being a dream.

The only true way of knowing is to have an etheric projection while awake, then you will know the difference.

This is the exact same experience that one has when they have a near death experience. Your energy lifts out of the body and usually hovers over it, watching all the goings on below.

The difference between a near death experience, or etheric projection, and an actual death is that the energy has not completely detached from the physical body and has no intention of detaching. Rather they are simply experiencing being out of it for a short period of time. It is much more common than people realize.

I find it fascinating to hear about the many books on the market today that talk about people's near death experiences and how amazing they are, more amazing still is that their readers think it is absolutely amazing.

In truth, it is very common and is a natural part of our lives. To experience it consciously, rather than while asleep, is what makes it different to some.

In discussing etheric projection with people that have claimed to have near death experiences, they soon realize one thing, that a part of their energy was still attached to the body. This is often overlooked as so many people believe that they have actually died and come back. This is not the case at all. They have never truly taken all of the energy out of the body nor have they completely severed from it. If they had then they would not come back.

When you have an etheric projection, or a near death experience if you prefer to call it, there is a thin rope of lighted energy that is attaching you and your physical body. This thin rope of energy is attached from the back of your neck area when you are out of the body and attached to the physical body, usually around the solar plexus. This is called the Life Force area.

When someone experiences a sudden car crash or shock of some kind, their energy can easily be bumped or jolted out of the physical body and they find themselves floating above. If they were to pay close attention, they would soon notice a thin rope of energy that extends upwards from the physical body below. Unfortunately most people experiencing an etheric projection are too fascinated with how they feel and what is happening to their body beneath them that they do not notice or pay attention to the thin rope of lighted energy. If they do, they only notice it floating upwards and do not realize that it is attached to the backs of their own neck area.

This ropy light is actually feeding the body enough energy to sustain it until you are ready to re-enter it. This too has aroused much confusion with people.

Some have wrongly believed that the rope of lighted energy is holding you, the spirit, down to the body, so that you don't float away into infinite space and death. This then creates a fear in people that somehow that line of lighted energy is delicate and can be broken or even cut by some unknown source, wherein you can't get back in. Fantasies always lead to fearful speculation and unfortunately causes people to fear out of body experiences.

In actuality, you, the spirit, are attaching your energy to the body and keeping it alive, not the other way around. The body is not holding you, you are holding and sustaining the body. The reason being is that you are not finished with it yet. During a past life regression death memory you experience something quite different because you are actually leaving the body for good. There is no chord or rope of lighted energy at all, because you have decided not to keep the body going in case you change your mind.

The fear that some other spirit force can come along and disconnect you from your body, causing you to be a lost spirit forever, is quite ridiculous. Only you can decide when to sever from your body, no one else. No one can cut the chord but you. When you are ready to die you do not create any chord at all. You only create a chord of lighted energy attaching you to the body when you are planning to have an etheric projection.

I say this because of the use of the term near death experience. I don't believe a person who has jolted out of the body is actually near death at all, but simply jolted out of their body, which is an etheric projection and a common occurrence.

Death was never the intention, but more likely a learning about oneself and an opportunity to experience being out of the body while conscious rather than asleep, which is what most people do.

If every out of body experience were considered to be a near death experience, then we would be having near death experiences almost nightly. So it is not such an amazing experience after all, but one that is very common and natural.

You can experiment in small ways with your energy to get a feel for what it is like to have an etheric projection. Simply lie still for at least half an hour with no pillow and then focus your attention on your feet. Feel as though they are becoming longer and longer. You will soon actually feel your feet extending, even to the point of feeling the edge of the bed. You can do the same with your hands, only this time focus on raising your hand. Soon you will feel your hand floating above your actual physical hand, which has not moved.

Scientific minds will say this is simply imagination. But if you keep practicing, soon you will find yourself floating completely above your body and around the room, and, eventually to visit other people where you can watch them discussing the days events. Afterwards, you can tell them what they were discussing and they will wonder how you knew.

Etheric projection is certainly not a subject that is new in the world. Much has been written about it and many experiments by many logically focussed minds, such as doctors and psychologists, have studied and researched it. Unfortunately, they do not usually understand the difference between the mind astral layer and the etheric layer, as they do not realize there are any layers at all and they lump everything together.

This is also what people do when it comes to death experiences and astral projections, as well as etheric projections. They lump everything together and believe that all are the same and the only difference is that when you die you just keep on going.

Actually, when you die you are moving onto a different layer of the Astral or Bardo realm altogether. The third layer.

This third layer is what I call the Ghost level. I think it is important once and for all to understand what is really happening when it comes to ghosts.

When a spirit decides to leave its body for good with the death experience, they move immediately into the third level of the Astral or Bardo realm. They move through two dimensional layers, the mind astral and the etheric and go immediately to the third, the Ghost level.

This layer of the Astral dimension is very close to our own dimension, it is only separated by a few thin veils of vibrational energy.

When a being lifts from their body during death they move into this layer and they usually look down upon the body they have just left. They will not have a lighted energy chord attached to the body. They have taken all of their energy completely out and the body cannot be restored because the spirit has completely severed itself from the body. The body might as well be a piece of furniture as far as the spirit is concerned, as it has no connection to it any longer.

When a spirit leaves its body for good and immediately moves to this level, it will often linger there for a while. It must be understood that now that it has completely severed itself from the body it is no longer attached to the illusion of time. It floats above the body for a brief moment but then quickly searches for the loved ones that it has left behind.

The spirit lingers here and usually tries to connect with those left behind in order to assure them that they are fine and still close by. Unfortunately, most people cannot perceive them and miss the opportunity of connecting with the spirit.

If a person can get beyond their grief, they are usually surprised that they can sense the presence of their dead loved one. The spirit will often try very hard to get the attention of those in the body and often does. It will swirl around people sometimes, even move objects, which takes a great deal of effort for the spirit. The reason the spirit does this is to comfort loved ones, not to frighten them.

Unfortunately, most people's beliefs about spirits gets in the way and they become fearful if they sense the presence of a spirit.

A spirit will usually only linger in this space for a short while, according to our time frame, as it is longing to move onwards. This is why people will usually sense the presence of a dead loved one for a period of a few weeks to a few months, then suddenly it is gone.

The reason for this is that the spirit is being enticed by a beautifully loving and brilliantly lit, presence. Its higher self. Whenever one leaves the body, even in an etheric projection, one is aware of a loving light nearby. One's higher self is always there in the Astral or Bardo realm and is always willing to commune with you.

If you are a regular practitioner of deep meditation you will experience a union with your higher self, which creates an incredible bliss within you. Joining with one's higher self is the most loving experience possible. Much more loving than one can experience with a human.

When you die, however, your higher self is most eager to reunite with you and to fill you with love and a sense of wholeness once again. Remember this is also possible to experience in an out of body journey or in deep meditation, but not as completely as when we free ourselves from the body through death.

Your higher self longs to move you onwards to a place of peace and to detach you from associating with your past for too long. You have just been through a life experience of being separate from your higher self and alone and so it is time for you to re-experience a pure love and wholeness that can only come from your other half, your higher self.

Usually, the spirit is most willing to quickly move away from its relatives and enter the brilliant loving light that awaits them. Sometimes a spirit will not stay at all as it recognizes that no one will be able to sense it anyway so why bother, or it feels no great connection to anyone left behind. It then immediately joins with the higher self as soon as it lifts from the body.

There is on occasion, however, a rare occurrence. A spirit that wants to linger close to those still in physical bodies. This is what is commonly called a ghost or astral spirit. Most often a spirit will move quickly through this level and onto the next.

When a spirit decides to stay on this level it is usually because it is unaware that it is dead and it is trying to communicate with those still in a body.

This happens when a being is jolted out of a body suddenly as in a car accident or sudden death. They find themselves floating above their body and unaware of what just happened. Because of their confusion they are also unwilling to recognize or pay attention to the loving light of their higher self, which is trying to get their attention.

Instead, they focus on their body, which they find beneath them, and when the body does not respond, they move to other people, who are actively moving about. They will then focus their attention on trying to communicate with those people and can do so for an unlimited amount of time.

It is important to remember that this recently deceased spirit is no longer in time. This is why is it a common occurrence for people to hear about or see a ghostly spirit that seems to be walking around a castle in England, for instance, and it seems to be about three hundred years old.

People then begin to think, "How horrible. That spirit has been walking in this state for three hundred years. What a torture."

This is not the case, however. To that spirit, it has just died because it is no longer in time as we are. To us, three hundred years may have passed, but according to that spirit, it has just died.

Everything is "now" when you are out of the body. A concept that I realize is hard to grasp but can be experienced by having an etheric projection. Then you will understand as you will feel that a moment has passed and when you come back to your body and look at the clock, hours may have passed.

What needs to be understood, however, is why the spirit has chosen to linger in this third layer of the Astral or Bardo realm.

Contrary to the belief of most horror movie addicts and writers, it is not to torment us and frighten us to death. It is actually to find understanding by trying to communicate with someone in a body.

Put yourself in the place of the spirit. It has just been bumped out of its body by some event and doesn't understand what happened. It's higher self, a beautiful loving light is trying to get its attention, but the spirit wants to know what just happened as it still feels alive. So what to do? Why not try and communicate with some of those people wandering around down on the planet? Seems like a good idea!

So the spirit lingers in the third layer and tries to communicate with those still in bodies. Sometimes it succeeds, sometimes it frightens people, depending on the perception of the human it is trying to communicate with.

What it does not do, however, is try to hurt people or terrorize them to death. There would be absolutely no reason for this.

The idea of evil spirits is one invented by people trying to control others by instilling fear, or by malicious ego-maniacal, power hungry personalities, of which there are many in the world. Those few people in the world that have died after seeing a spirit have died because of their own fear, not because of the spirit.

I have in my career come across numerous spirits lingering in the third level, as people seem to feel it necessary to call me when they find one. I am then amazed to hear of how the spirit is tormenting them by moving objects around. Their version is that the spirit is trying to kill them or get them to move out of the house. The spirit is moving objects in order to get the person's attention, not to terrorize them. Fear again, supersedes common sense.

If a person sees or senses the presence of a ghost, or astral spirit as I prefer to call them, it is much wiser to try to communicate. If they are perceptive enough to sense the spirit, then maybe they can also be of help to that spirit.

How to help a confused spirit? Tell it that it is dead and it must now move on to its light. Tell it to move to its higher self and to complete with its past life. Tell it that its higher self will help it to understand its past life but that you cannot.

Amazingly, the spirit leaves. Simple isn't it, yet something that people rarely think of doing. Instead people run away in terror. Imagine how the spirit must feel when everyone runs away? How would you feel?

A number of years ago a friend of mine and I went into the basement of an old restaurant in Vancouver where it had been well known that the spirit of a child had been heard crying for decades. Numerous restaurants had also failed while inhabiting the premises and so the spirit was blamed. The poor spirit. Imagine blaming the failure of a restaurant on a spirit. Could it have been possible that the restaurants would have failed anyway? Is it not common for many restaurants to last only a few years? No one thought of that, however. Blame it on the spirit. Maybe the tax department would give them a special write-off procedure for "Bankruptcy by Ghost!"

When my friend and I entered the basement, we spent some time sitting quietly and asking the spirit if it would be willing to allow us to help it. Soon after we both felt the presence of the spirit sitting in the corner of the hallway. It felt like a small boy child. Neither my friend nor I saw it, but only felt it.

I then began to hear a vague voice calling "Where's mommy?" over and over again. I asked the spirit if it could show me what happened and then maybe I could help.

We then began to vaguely smell smoke and I began to see, although extremely hazily, a fire erupting through the entire building, although the building I was seeing was not the same as the present one. I then saw a young woman crying out for her child and then fall, after which I saw a young boy running through the flames crying out for his mother, who I presumed was already dead. The boy then also died, but somehow his spirit was not willing to admit this and was insisting on continuing the search for his mother. This was the ghostly presence that everyone had been hearing for many years. This child calling out for his mommy.

My friend and I felt heartbroken but realized that we must tell this spirit that its mother had died and that he too, must move on now. We encouraged it to look to the light that was behind it and to move towards it and let go the search for his mother.

We did this by talking aloud to the spirit. Some people may think we were mad to think we could communicate with the spirit, or that it would care to listen to us, but it did. It immediately left and we felt a sudden emptiness in the hallway.

It took very little effort or bravery on our part, simply a few words of encouragement and direction, something anyone can give to a confused spirit. Fear is simply a projection in our minds created by watching too many horror movies. To have an opportunity to help a spirit is truly an honor and I have felt blessed in being able to do so.

I also had the experience of having a woman bring her 12 year old son to visit me. She explained to me that since the age of one there were spirits floating around him in his room and they would do horrific things which she wanted stopped.

When I asked what the horrific things were she told me that they would raise his body and would toss his toys around the room. She explained how terrified she had been on numerous occasions to enter her young son's room only to find him floating above his crib. She made it sound like a scene from The Exorcist.

As I listened to the woman's terrible tales of woe, I noticed that the young man was sitting quietly and looking out of my window, as though completely uninterested in what she was saying.

I interrupted the woman and asked her son how he felt about the spirits. He looked startled and then turned to his mother who quickly replied, "Well of course he wants them to leave, he's afraid of them too. Who knows what they might do next? I'm afraid for his life."

At this expression of worry, I noticed a slight sly smile on the boy's face and I realized that more was going on here than the mother knew.

Over the years, whenever I had come across someone who was having numerous experiences with an astral spirit, I was surprised to find that they had often, not always, but often unconsciously invited that spirit to come into their lives. I had the inclination that this was the case with this young man as well.

I again asked the son directly how he felt about the spirits. He gave me a quizzical look, as though he was suddenly discovered harboring a great secret. He hesitated and his mother nudged him to reply, to which he replied that he liked them.

Needless to say his mother was astonished and immediately chastised him for saying such a ridiculous thing. She also told him point blank that, "Of course he doesn't like them."

I then asked the mother to be quiet for a moment as I talked directly to him and encouraged him to be completely honest with me. I asked him if he truly wanted the spirits to leave. He became edgy and fidgeted in his chair as he replied that he did not want them to leave because they were his friends.

To make a long story short, the boy had invited these spirits to come and be his playmates when he was a baby because he had no father around and his mother was continually away at work. As he grew, his neighborhood friends would come over and the spirits would move objects around the room, causing this young man to be the center of attention in the neighborhood and at school. He became very popular because of his astral spirit friends and he certainly did not want them to leave.

Often small children can see spirits in the form of colored spheres of energy. As they grow they become involved in the world around them and they lose this vision. If you question small children, you will be amazed at what they can see. Often they can also see auric fields around people. I have had a number of small children tell me about the purple color they were seeing around me.

After a long discussion with the young man and his mother, I told him that he had the power to ask the spirits to leave and only he had that power, as they had come to be with him and only when he was ready to say goodbye would they leave.

But why would an astral spirit linger in such a state, I questioned to myself? I could only reason that the spirits must have been a part of the boy's soul family and had agreed to linger in the third level of the astral realm in order to assist a loved one. Since they were not connected to time any longer, it certainly didn't matter to them how long it took before he chose to say goodbye. I didn't hear back from them, so I don't know how it ended.

Once you have completed with the astral spirit level it is time to rejoin with the higher self and the fourth level - the Higher Self level.

As explained earlier, this is a unification of immense love and oneness, a totality of being that cannot be readily understood while still in a body. You can only re-experience the memory of it while in a past life regression.

The fifth level is the Examination of Life level where one takes the opportunity to look back into the past and truly examine it all thoroughly. It is here that you realize what your lessons had been and if you had actually learned them all or not. It is common during a regression to realize here that you did not actually fulfill your lessons completely and so you will want to do so in a future life.

This is the level one returns to in a regression to complete the healing and to understand the past life.

The sixth level is the rest period, which was explained previously and is simply a time to rest.

The seventh level is called the level of Choice and is the final level of the Astral or Bardo realm before one returns to the body and begins the whole procedure all over again. This is where one chooses one's parents and basic blueprint for the life to come. This is also the level where one hovers over the left shoulder of the mother during the nine month period of pregnancy.

CHAPTER SEVENTEEN

Soul Mates, Soul Family And Essence Twins

EVERY SINCE I CAN REMEMBER I have been hearing about soul mates. People seem to go through their lives endlessly searching for their soul mate. That perfect person who is so compatible with you that you will join together in ultimate bliss and have the perfect relationship, filled with strawberries and cream and never, ever, have an argument.

Sound like a romantic fantasy movie? I think so. Have you ever met anyone personally that had such a relationship? Probably never. That is because it is an unrealistic fantasy, which has been created by romantics who long to believe that perfect relationships mean no conflict.

Your soul mate is said to be so in sync with you that you love to do the same things together and you have everything the same in common, you love the same food, etc., and sex is absolutely amazing. It is also said that your soul mate is, being so like you, so easy to recognize because of the similarities.

Unfortunately when you meet someone who is so similar to yourself and has everything in common with you, there is usually something missing. That illusive spark or chemistry that draws people to one another.

Have you ever heard the term, "Opposite's Attract?" Well it's true, opposites do attract each other. The reason being is that being with someone who is so like yourself is usually boring. It is like looking in the mirror. Rarely when we meet someone like this is there passion, electricity or compatibility. You become tired of each other very quickly if your mate is too similar to you.

Over the years I have talked to so many woman and men who are still seeking their soul mate. Unfortunately because of this seeking, they keep passing up wonderful relationships with people who come into their lives, because they believe that the person is too different from themselves, and, therefore, could not possibly be their soul mate.

Relationships are about growth, as is the purpose of existence on this planet. Therefore, looking for a mate that is so similar to yourself, is looking to create a dead relationship.

It is very hard to grow when you are in a boring relationship and what usually happens is you start looking for more exciting people and relationships because your soul mate is boring you to tears.

The truth is your soul mate or mates are not similar to you at all. Who is? Your Essence Twin.

An Essence Twin is a spirit who is evolving at a similar pace to your own and who has spent numerous lives with you. Your growth pattern is similar and you come into each other's lives over and over again to help each other by being supportive and offering advice and comfort. An Essence Twin does not make a good partner for a relationship however, and this is where confusion arises.

Usually an Essence Twin will show up in our lives in the form of a best friend or even a parent. They have the same likes and dislikes and sometimes are so similar in personality that you try to make a relationship out of the friendship.

An Essence Twin is someone who is there for you, who understands your woes and who listens attentively. Someone you can count on. Often there is a desire to spend a great deal of time with an Essence Twin because of your similar likes.

What is not a good idea is to try to turn an Essence Twin relationship into an intimate one. It never works because their is no electricity between the two of you.

I went through this experience with a man when I was in my twenties. We immediately had a lot in common and felt very close to each other.

Unfortunately, when we moved the friendship to an intimate one, it felt very strange and their was no spark or chemistry.

You are also usually psychically connected to an Essence Twin and this is another reason why people try to turn the relationship into an intimate one. They believe that a person can only be truly psychically connected with a soul mate. Not true. An Essence Twin is much more likely to be in tune to your thoughts and desires.

Another problem with turning an Essence Twin relationship into an intimate one is that it is often uncomfortable having someone know you so well and be so like you. They are always showing you every aspect of yourself. This is fine in a friendship and can be extremely helpful in your growth, which is what an Essence Twin relationship is for, growth and support. But in an intimate relationship it usually causes frustration to continually be the same as the person you are intimate with.

During my life I have experienced another Essence Twin relationship with a woman friend and it was fascinating to discover how similar we were. We used to joke that we were really the same person split into two bodies. We both sang opera and would undergo very similar changes and thought patterns. We would finish each other's sentences and when one of us would have a craving, the other would often go out and buy the food, not knowing why.

What I found interesting about the relationship and what I have discovered in my research of other Essence Twin relationships, is that there is great joy in spending time together and discussing various life experiences, but it is uncomfortable to spend long periods of time together.

This was my own experience. I longed to be with my friend but I found that if I were to spend more than a few days together, I couldn't wait to get away. It was like constantly analyzing your own life and psyche. It is certainly helpful in understanding yourself, but to continue it hour after hour for days is very tiring and soon becomes boring as well.

We seem to need to be around people that are different from ourselves in order to stretch ourselves and grow. If we only spend time around those that are very similar, there is little, or no growth. You can spend time analyzing each other, but only by understanding and being with different people, do we truly grow.

In other words, with an Essence Twin, it is almost like being in a mutual admiration society. You continually praise each other because if you don't then you are criticizing yourself. Unfortunately, with continual praise, there tends to be an unwillingness to see truth.

This is why it feels so good to go to your best friend or Essence Twin when you have a fight with your mate. Your Essence Twin is always on your side, because you think the same way. It feels wonderful to be supported by your Essence Twin, but it doesn't help you to see the other side of the situation. Your Essence Twin will only see your side, which is often what you want.

I find it fascinating to hear how people who are in arguments go and spend time with their best friend, who completely agrees with them, only to return to their relationship and say, "Well so and so agrees with me, so I must be right."

Your Essence Twin helps you to justify your actions and behavior but it must be realized that they do that only because they are so similar.

Some people then say to me, "well wouldn't that make a great relationship then, both of you would think the same, so there would be no conflict". That's true, there would be no conflict, but there would be no passion or growth either.

I have known a few people who have been in a married relationship with an Essence Twin and they speak of how the relationship is so peaceful and calm, and of how similar they are. Yet, when I speak to them individually about the relationship, they always speak about there being something missing. They're not sure what it is and they convince themselves that they couldn't ask for a better relationship, but still, inside they are longing for more passion, fire or something intense.

I have found that people in an intimate relationship with an Essence Twin will eventually look for something to argue about, even ridiculous things, just to bring some spark into the relationship. In time, the women usually turn to reading romance novels about passion and excitement and the men turn to sports.

The relationship then has little or no growth in it and the two turn to other things or relationships to stimulate them. Boredom in a relationship is death. We must inspire and stir each other in order to grow and stop trying to be the same.

So enjoy the time spent with Essence Twins and forget trying to turn the friendship into a relationship. As far as waiting for your perfect soul mate, stop waiting and start living, now.

As far as the term soul mate, meaning one mate, is concerned, I don't believe that it truly exists either. We have been taught to believe that we have one soul mate in our life and if we happen to miss each other, well too bad, we just end up being alone.

In truth, we have many soul mates who are a part of an extended soul family.

Our soul family is comprised of a vast number of spirits, which can range from twenty to more than a hundred, with whom we reincarnate over and over again. We do this in order to help each other evolve and to learn and create karmic experiences together. We need to form connections with a great number of spirits in order to create experiences together. For instance, our father in one life may become our child in another, in order to learn about both experiences and to teach each other different things.

We have come to this planet to learn everything it has to offer about the human experience and so we keep bumping into spirits who are doing the same thing and we agree to help each other grow. This is why there is a feeling of knowing certain people before. You have, and probably many times.

We need to have a large soul family because we keep moving around the planet and turning up in different places with different cultures. We may have spent numerous lives in say, Europe, but now we have decided to be born in the United States because one of our soul family has journeyed there and we want to be born into their family in our new life.

Sometimes you can feel an unusual sensation with someone in your soul family. For instance, you may feel very paternal to your mother or father or to a sister or friend. This feeling is being carried forward in your memory from when you were perhaps the parent and they the child.

For instance, I had always felt very motherly to my own father in this life. When he used to drink I would completely revert to being his mother and even send him to his room. It never even seemed amazing to me that he would immediately obey, without question. Unconsciously he was responding to me as my child as well and went to his room quietly. Most of the time I felt much older than him and I was always very worried about him and wanted to take care of him.

This is actually quite a common experience and one that is easily understood by doing a past life regression and then remembering where it was that you had experienced such a relationship before. I came to realize that I had been a mother to my present father numerous times and so it was natural for me to react as a mother around him and to care for him, even to chastise him when he would drink heavily.

As we have many other beings in our soul family, it is from within this extended family that we will choose mates. Not one mate that we continually join with in intimacy over and over again, but many mates.

95

We are emotionally connected to all in our soul family and we will choose first to join with someone who happens to be in a body and, second, who will best help us to learn and grow and experience intimacy.

So the idea of having one and only one soul mate is ridiculous. If you are in a relationship with someone and it ends, there is more than a possibility of having another mate in your life.

CHAPTER EIGHTEEN

Hypnosis

HYPNOSIS WAS DEVELOPED BY A man named Mr. Mesmer in the 18th century and used to be called mesmerizing. It's the act of focusing the mind within and distancing oneself from outer sounds and events while at the same time relaxing the body. The hypnotist uses his/her voice to create an inner focus in the subject. The patient is totally alert and awake, not unconscious as many people believe. Nor do they forget everything afterwards.

There are two different types of hypnosis. Stage hypnosis and self-hypnosis, both of which use the sympathetic and para-sympathetic nervous systems. However, the similarities end there.

To understand hypnosis one must understand what is happening to the brain.

The brain vibrates on frequencies or oscillations. This is the speed at which the brain is functioning. We have heard about the four basic oscillations, which are Beta, Alpha, Theta and Delta. However, there is one more, which has not, to my knowledge, been given a name. This is the frequency which is above Beta and which is used by stage hypnotists.

The stage hypnotist is moving the brain's oscillations to a higher speed, which makes it difficult for most people to understand what is happening to them. To begin, the hypnotist will keep people on the stage that are excited. This means that the brain's oscillations are becoming faster as the person becomes excited. For most people, being called up on a stage in front of thousands of people and having bright lights beaming into their eyes causes some excitement and nervousness to say the least. If a person comes onto the stage who is very relaxed, the hypnotist will tell them to go and sit down. The hypnotist only wants those people who are becoming excited or nervous, which can easily be detected.

The hypnotist will then usually talk to the person a while and encourage their nervousness even more. At this point the brain has gone from Beta to a higher level of oscillation. In other words, it is speeding up.

Then the hypnotist will do a variety of different things depending on their technique. Often they will have the person close their eyes and the hypnotist will make a loud clap beside their head which encourages the brain to move even faster because the person is in unfamiliar surroundings and knows they are being watched. Then the hypnotist will usually touch the person firmly somewhere around the temple or head. This thrusts the brain's oscillations into hyper-mode. At this point the person is aware but unable to reason or make choices. The person is in reactive-mode and will respond to almost anything. Why? Because the speed of the brain makes it difficult, if not impossible, for the person to understand what is happening. The hypnotist then asks them to bark like a dog and what happens? They respond, without question. They are in a simple reactive mode because their brain is moving too fast for them to make sense of what is being asked of them. So they simply respond to the suggestion.

If they were in a situation where they were relaxed and the brain's oscillations actually slowed down, then they would easily be able to reason that it is not really a good idea for them to bark like a dog and so they would refuse.

This type of hypnosis has no benefits except to entertain and in my opinion, is not a healthy type of entertainment. It is a way of using people and belittling them. However, what we can learn from the situation is how the brain works and how hypnosis works.

This form of hypnosis is not the standard hypnosis used in regression therapy or any other type of healing therapy.

Something very important can be learned from the type of hypnosis used by stage entertainers. The brain is the inhibitor, not the source, to wisdom and memory.

If the brain were the source of wisdom and memory, then we should assume that the faster the oscillations of the brain, which means the more active the brain is, the smarter we should be, right? Not so. The more active the brain, the less we are able to comprehend and process.

On the contrary, the slower the oscillations of brain, the more memory and wisdom we receive and reveal.

Proof of this is quite simple. How often have you tried, in vain, to remember someone's name or perhaps a place? You force and push and try with all of your might to remember, but it eludes you. You feel as though it is on the tip of your tongue but you can't quite find it.

That is because by trying to remember, you are actually speeding up the brain's oscillations, which makes it more difficult to remember or process thought or wisdom.

Then something wonderful happens. You go to bed and you relax, or you wake up and are relaxed and suddenly, without effort, you remember what you could not remember earlier. It's right there and you are amazed at how you could have possibly forgotten.

What has happened is that the brain's oscillations have slowed to an Alpha level when you are relaxed and near sleep or have just awoken and the brain is no longer blocking your memories.

Writers and all creative people experience the same thing. I have spoken with many writers who complain about writer's block. They sit in front of their word processor and they try and try to come up with something but cannot. Then they go to bed at night and suddenly a great flood of words comes pouring through them.

If you speak with writer's or artists or even a business person who has been struggling with an idea of some sort, they will tell you that they are most creative at night, when they are relaxed. In other words, when the brain's oscillations are slowed down to an Alpha, or even a Theta level.

This understanding of the brain is very important because medical science has always taught us to believe that the brain is the source of our wisdom and memory. I disagree. I believe that the brain is the tool with which we bring that information through to form words and language to intellectualize or share with the outside world, but that it is not the source. It is in fact, the barrier.

A case in fact is Ginny, a young woman who came to me in 1989. She had experienced some brain damage in a car accident two years earlier and had lost the memories of her childhood from before the age of ten.

Now the scientist would argue with me that because Ginny lost brain cells in the accident, she therefore lost memory and it could not be restored. I questioned that.

Indeed Ginny had lost brain cells which made it difficult for her to process her memory through the brain but the memories were not destroyed because the memories are not stored in the brain cells, they are stored in the energy which is at the core of the brain cell.

Quantum energy as science calls it, is what makes up each cell and so it is the energy that carries the memories, not the cell itself. Science also has proven that energy cannot be destroyed, it can only change form, so the energy that had stored Ginny's memories had not been destroyed, it had simply changed from being within those cells to being another part of her energy formation.

To find Ginny's memories, I needed to slow down the speed of her brain in order to allow her memories to resurface. What Ginny had previously being trying to do was to force herself to remember her past by pushing or trying. She did this by looking at pictures and talking to relatives. Unfortunately her brain was in the way. By relaxing her and slowing the oscillations of the brain, Ginny's childhood memories resurfaced just as they had been before, without alteration of any kind, and now she was able to bring those memories through her current brain cells and see them whenever she wanted as well as talk about them.

Everything has a purpose in our existence and I believe the brain does as well, but not for the function most people believe. I believe that it is an inhibitor to our past memories in order to protect us from remembering everything about our past lives.

If we were to come into a body with full memory of all of our past lives, it would be very difficult to create a new experience in our present body. We would be hounded by our past mistakes, fears and personalities.

We need to create a form of amnesia when we begin a new life in order to start afresh and learn a new experience with our fresh new bodies. If we were fully conscious of all of our past lives it would be a lot of baggage to carry, especially through our youth.

So our brain helps us to create a barrier to our past memories, but not a barrier so strong that it cannot be penetrated. By using past life regression and relaxing hypnosis, we are able to slow down the brain's protective speed and allow our memories to resurface.

Even though our brain is an inhibitor, some past life memories and certainly issues from our past lives that have been unresolved seem to seep to the surface to be healed in the present.

Often past life memories surface in our dreams, as we are in an Alpha state of awareness.

When we are children, our most recent past life also often resurfaces. This is because children's brains are often relaxed and they are not straining. Also because they have most recently come from a previous life, the memories can still be quite fresh. Unfortunately, the more they grow, the more they forget, as they are using their brains far more frequently by learning in school. The relaxed state of being is replaced by pressure and stress.

I have often had parents bring me their children or write to me about their child's experiences of past life memories. One particular time in London, England when I did a live television talk show with a phone in question and answer session, a woman told me of her young daughter who had begun to speak French before her native English. The family was naturally astounded as none of them spoke French. Still they passed it off as her having watched too much television.

When the child was near four, she began to talk about her other mommy and daddy and her other sisters. She told her stunned mother about how they used to do the washing before and she described in great detail, an antique type of washing basin. She also went on to describe her other house where she lived with her other mommy and daddy.

Needless to say, her mother was shocked and disturbed by her young daughter's words and when she called the television show she was anxious to find help.

I told her what I tell all parents of young children. That it is perfectly natural for young children to remember their past lives and it is important to encourage them, not to stifle them or tell them that they are making it up. This is what many parents do and soon the children learn that it is not safe to express their true feelings and they learn to cover up and forget their memories.

Eventually the memories will fade into the distant past anyway as they create a new personality and knowledge again. However, the memories are not gone, they are temporarily forgotten as they have no use at the present time and can often create confusion in the child.

In time, as the child ages and becomes an adult, past life memories often resurface, but usually only those that require a balancing or healing.

Sometimes a past life memory will resurface in the form of what we call "Deja Vu". This is a sense or feeling that we have been in a certain place before or that it feels familiar. This is because it is familiar.

People have told me of their experiences in Europe for instance, where they were simply walking around the streets shopping when suddenly an overwhelming feeling of having been there before comes over them. They can often remember what is around the next corner and will sometimes vaguely see visions of people in ancient dress walking about in front of them.

This experience happened to me quite by surprise when I was visiting London, England. A friend of mine decided to show me some sights nearby and we ended up walking amidst a beautiful old ruin of an ancient castle. The gardens and grounds were beautiful but there was little left of any buildings, just some occasional stone walls and walkways where there had been buildings.

It was a beautiful and warm sunny day as we strolled amongst the grounds when I suddenly heard a distinct rustling sound. I stopped and asked my friend if he had heard it and he replied that he hadn't heard anything. Surprised at his answer, I decided to forget it and continue. We strolled a little further and I heard the rustling sound again. This time it was even clearer and I was sure my friend must of heard it that time. He again replied that he didn't. I explained to him that it sounded like heavy fabric rustling. Within moments of continuing our walk, I began to actually feel myself walking differently as I became aware that I felt as though I were wearing a heavy, long dress with a tight bodice.

As we walked, my senses became clearer and I could actually vaguely see this dress that I was wearing. It was a silver brocaded gown with embroidery on the bodice and sleeves. I also felt myself to be much shorter and more petite.

This became a fascinating experience and we continued walking slowly as the vision and hearing senses began to unfold even further.

I started to tell my friend various things about myself, such as my name and why I was there when suddenly I could see the castle as it must have been.

Although the vision was vague, it was clear enough for me to see some intricate details.

I told my friend that I was a guest in this castle and I was here for a wedding. No sooner had I told him this than I began to hear muttering sounds to my right. I turned around and was amazed as a picture unfolded in front of me.

I saw across the courtyard numerous ladies and gentlemen, all dressed in early sixteenth century finery walking about the gardens, which were much more lush and beautiful.

I explained to my friend that I felt as though I were a distant cousin to the woman about to be married here and I felt very honored and excited to be a part of the whole affair.

This past life vision lasted for about ten minutes and then faded just as quickly as it had come.

Afterwards, I felt completely amazed and excited as I had never experienced such a thing before. However, during my research over the years about past life regression, I had heard about many instances of what was called "spontaneous regression". This is obviously what I had experienced.

During my research, I came to learn that the more one undergoes past life regression under hypnosis, the more one is likely to experience a spontaneous regression because one is regularly opening the memory banks.

Since regressing thousands of people and discussing the subject with many more during conventions and on television and radio, I have realized that it is not such an uncommon experience after all.

Many people have told me of spontaneous regression visions that they have experienced, but more often than not, they were surprised and confused by the vision and immediately stopped it by thinking about something else.

Unfortunately, fear of the unknown commonly stops people from experiencing their past.

After I had my experience in London, I began to reflect on it and I soon remembered an experience I had as a young woman.

I had been resting on my side on the couch in the living room watching the springtime sun shining through the windows and making patterns on the carpet. I was relaxed and peaceful and simply enjoying the afternoon. I was not asleep and certainly not dreaming. I lay there propped up against the side of the couch with my head resting on a pillow when I began to feel different. Without moving my head, I looked down towards my legs as I felt as though I were wearing heavier fabric.

To my surprise I could see myself wearing a heavily fabriced dark green/ brown dress.

Again without moving, I noticed the room seemed to change as I looked at it. The walls took on a vague look of wooden walls and the room seemed to be smoky as the sun poured in.

What I remember about the experience was not so much the look of everything, but how I felt. I felt different, yet the same.

The most fascinating feeling, however, was that I had somehow found myself in a past experience, yet I was doing the exact same thing. I was laying on a type of settee in the same position and it felt as though I were doing the exact same thing. I was enjoying the afternoon sun entering the room and making a pattern on the carpet.

It is very difficult to describe my feelings at the time, but I was acutely aware that I was in another woman's body and yet I felt as though I were myself, in the present, as well. It was very confusing and after probably five minutes of the experience, it faded and I soon forgot about it because someone knocked on my door.

These experiences are what we call Deja Vu. In London I had been in the exact place that I had been once before and so the memory simply resurfaced without effort. If I had been busily talking or doing something, the memory very likely would not have surfaced, but because I was relaxed and quietly enjoying the walk amongst the gardens, the memory came alive. The same happened with the past experience on the couch. I was relaxed and peaceful and so the memory of doing the exact same thing in a past life resurfaced.

Deja vu does not mean you have to be in the exact same place, you can also simply be experiencing the same thing, when the past memory resurfaces.

In both of these above instances, my brain waves would have been slowed down to an Alpha level because I was relaxed and not thinking about anything, just enjoying the moment.

If I had been in a Beta brain awareness it would be unlikely I would have remembered anything at all.

Beta is the state of awareness that we are in during most of the day. When we are working, talking, interacting with others and functioning at a normal brain speed, we are in Beta.

The next level of the brain's oscillation is Alpha. This is one level lower than Beta and this is what most people will experience as anything from a quiet relaxed state to a deep relaxation, which you find yourself in just prior to sleep.

As you begin your sleep procedure you move from Beta, through Alpha, which is also where you dream, and into Theta.

When you are dreaming you are not actually in what I would call, sleep mode. You are close but certainly not in a deep sleep. You are on the surface level of sleep and dreams are very prominent there.

Although science has studied these levels of the brain's oscillations, I don't feel they have, as yet, understood the many layers within them.

Alpha, for instance, is not simply where we dream, for there is a beginning Alpha and a deeper Alpha, just before we move into Theta.

In other words, as we are slowing down our brain waves we first move into the top of Alpha and then deeper into it and then down to the bottom of Alpha and then finally into Theta.

Through my tests of the Alpha and Theta levels, I have come to realize that the top of Alpha is a relaxed state with complete awareness. What you feel when you go to bed and begin to relax. You are aware and still quite awake, but relaxed.

As you move deeper into Alpha, your body becomes more still and your breathing slower. Soon your awareness of your thoughts lessens. I do not mean that your thoughts stop, because they do not, but your awareness of them lessens.

You begin to feel distant from your bedroom and from noises and soon find yourself in the dream state. This is what I call, Lower Alpha.

As your relaxation deepens, you move from dreams into a deeper relaxation which is when you move into Theta. The dreams stop and you are in a light sleep. The brain's oscillations are still slowing down and moving you deeper into the Theta awareness where your sleep becomes more and more peaceful.

The final level of sleep is Delta. We only, on average, move into Delta for approximately one hour a night. This is an extremely deep sleep where the brain's oscillations are very slow. If you have ever experienced trying to wake someone up who simply does not respond, they are in Delta. Some people also rarely, if ever, experience Delta, as they never sleep deeply enough.

The levels of sleep patterns which the brain moves through are actually the same levels which one moves through during a hypnosis induced past life regression as well as in meditation.

In meditation, for instance, you are slowing down your brain waves through the same levels of Alpha and Theta only you are keeping yourself awake and alert.

This is the difficulty most people have with meditation. They fall asleep because their brain's oscillations are slowing down and they are not used to staying awake.

Meditation is a training of the awareness to stay alert and aware while slowing down the speed of the brain and thereby creating a deep inner peace with awareness.

Hypnosis is the same, at least the hypnosis used for healing.

Unlike what the stage hypnotists use, the hypnosis used for past life regression is self-hypnosis. This is a slowing of the brain's oscillations in order to allow the memories from the past to resurface.

I have often been asked by the medical profession if regression is not actually dreaming, because one is slowing the brain waves. It is not. Dreaming takes place in the Alpha state whereas past life regression memories are a little deeper. The memories surface on the top level of the Theta awareness, which is just slightly deeper than the Alpha, where we dream.

The difficulty of accessing the Theta awareness, therefore, is rather obvious. How to stay awake and slow down the brain's oscillations at the same time. The key is to have a therapist talk you down. If you try to slow down the brain's oscillations on your own, you will fall asleep, unless you are a practiced meditator who has trained yourself to stay alert. Most people have not and so are unable to move into a Theta awareness and stay awake. This is why most people do not readily remember their past lives.

As the past life memories can be accessed anywhere from the bottom level of Alpha through to the middle of Theta, it is common for people to have some memories surface during their lifetime. The difference with having a regression is to have a vivid recollection, rather than a vague one.

As I experienced in London, my memory was vague, although clear enough for me to still see some detail, it was not as clear as a full regression would be. The reason is because I was walking around the gardens and therefore, was not any deeper than possibly a middle Alpha wave.

Also, as a regular meditator for many years, I find it easy to slow my brain's oscillations and to relax even while walking about and interacting with people.

I have found as a regression therapist that there is a level of relaxation that one encounters during a regression that offers the person to receive very vivid past life memories, and even current life memories for that matter. This level is encountered just as the person shifts from the Alpha to the Theta.

How do I know when this happens? No, I don't have a scientific instrument attached to people's heads in order to measure their brain waves. The people show me themselves when they are there.

Have you ever experienced falling asleep at night when suddenly your body twitches? This twitch is a signal that you are moving through the lower levels of Alpha.

The first time I experienced this twitch was in the hospital when I was seventeen. I was in severe pain and the doctors could not figure out what was wrong with me. They were unable to examine me as I was hyperventilating and screaming with pain. The doctor needed to relax me so that he could examine me.

He sat beside me and took my hand in his. He then began to stroke my hand softly as he spoke to me in a gentle and quiet voice. He told me to breathe very shallow and to pant softly, which helped to ease the pain. He then asked me to close my eyes as he continued to gently stroke my hand. After about five minutes of his soft voice soothing me, I began to relax and the pain eased. Then I noticed that my hand twitched as he stroked it. Right after it twitched, he told me that now I was ready for him to examine me as my body was relaxed enough.

What I didn't realize at the time was that the good doctor was hypnotizing me. It worked. Although unlike the hypnosis you see on the stage, with self-hypnosis, you are aware and alert and you know perfectly well where you are and what is going on around you.

As I later began to practice and study hypnosis and past life regression, I was fascinated to see my clients twitching whenever they moved deeper.

Through practice and questioning people, I soon realized that once the person had experienced a slight twitch, they were more easily able to remember their past lives.

From there I also learned that by taking the person a little deeper into the Theta awareness, the regressions became clearer and much more vivid in both the visual senses and the emotional.

The key then, was first to watch for the twitch, which can be from a slight finger twitch to a whole leg twitch, then to relax them a little bit more.

For some people, moving into a regression can be difficult. Not because they are unable to remember their past lives, or because they are afraid, but because they tend to fall asleep.

I cannot count how many times I have begun to regress a person only to have a resounding snore fill the room within minutes. For this reason,

I usually encourage people who have never been regressed to first practice meditation regularly or at least be sure that they are able to stay awake while relaxed.

I have found that people who work in stressful, high activity jobs, often find a way to power nap or fall asleep immediately when their head hits the pillow. These people will find it difficult to experience a past life regression. They will first need to learn to stay awake while relaxing the body. This is an exercise that can easily be learned, but to unlearn it is difficult. Those that enjoy being able to lie down and immediately fall asleep within the first minute or so may not want to learn to stay alert whilst slowing down the brain waves.

That alertness tends to become more and more prominent the more you meditate and the more you do regressions. This has many benefits, such as experiencing deep meditations and deep inner peace, but not everyone wants that.

With regressions, like meditation, you create a greater awareness and alertness while in deeper levels of relaxation. The benefits to this is that it allows a greater flow of your creative energy to come to the surface.

Most meditators will agree that when you move deeper into the Theta state you will find an immense flow of wisdom and creativity pouring forth. What you do with that creative flow is up to you.

One rather common question that I get asked about hypnosis and past life regression is if there is a possibility that your personality will be overcome by one from the past and if your present personality will be lost.

This is not a possibility for the simple reason that during a regression you are remembering a past life memory, not reliving it. Although the memories can be very vivid and even emotional, and you can feel very much as though you are that person from the past, you are still aware that you are you and that you are undergoing a regression memory.

Past life regression using hypnosis is an act of remembering, not reliving. Hypnosis allows us the opportunity to relax the body and thus, the brain waves, which then allows the doorway to the past memories to be open. From there we allow ourselves to step into the past memories, feeling fully as though we are re-entering that ancient body and its thoughts. However, when this occurs we still have a sense of who we are in the present as well. It can be a feeling of a split personality.

You then have two choices. One is to have the memory from outside of the body, the other is to experience the memory from within the body.

Remembering it from within is regressing, whereas looking at the memory from a distance is a detached memory.

With regression, it is important to have the person feel themselves re-enter the actual physical body of their past, not simply to watch the lifetime from a distance. The reason for this is that it gives you an overwhelmingly personal connection which you cannot refute. You feel yourself in a different body and you feel the emotions and know the thoughts of that body and personality. This is what makes it so real.

If you were to just watch a vision of a past life going by in your mind, it would be easy to pass it off as a fantasy, but when you feel yourself in a completely different body, which moves and talks differently than your own, it is quite difficult to convince yourself that it isn't real.

During my research of past life regression I have also come to realize that it is very difficult, if not impossible, to make up a past life. The memories flow with ease and with a pattern, unlike dreams or fantasies. The memories are also slow in movement, just as in life.

When I tried to encourage people to create something in their imagination while in a Theta state of relaxation, they would find themselves blank and unable to, or they would fall asleep.

During an Alpha state, however, they found it much more easy to make up a story. Thus, it is during an Alpha state that we find ourselves more creative.

When you move deeper into a Theta state it is difficult to create something that is unknown. For instance, a story. The Theta state seems to be an opening to a door of not only our past memories, but wisdom as well. Not knowledge, wisdom.

Often meditators will speak about moving into a deep meditation or Theta state and receiving floods of wisdom about the meaning of life and their purpose in the body as well as visions and memories of their past lives. However, they find it next to impossible to create something themselves out of thin air.

It is as though moving into a Theta state is tapping into your higher self. The wisdom and memories that come from this deep place are either a culmination of all of our past lives or are coming from our higher source. I believe they come from both. By moving aside the blockage of the brain, we open ourselves to receive both universal wisdom from our higher selves and the memories of our past lives. When we then escalate our brain waves and move upwards through the Alpha level, I find we are more able to utilize that wisdom and to create with it.

It is important to understand here that during the Theta state we are simply receivers, not doers. Yet when we elevate to an Alpha level we can create with the wisdom we have just received. Unfortunately, however, the more we escalate the brain's oscillations from that point, the less we are able to utilize the wisdom we received during the Theta state. In other words, when your brain waves move faster as in a Beta state or perhaps the level higher, which the stage hypnotists use, we find it more and more difficult to be creative.

I have gone over this because it is commonly argued by the scientific community that people remembering past lives are just making it up. That, like a dream, it can be created. This is just not true and I challenge anyone in a Theta state to be able to create a story with just their imagination that would make any sense whatsoever.

So often whilst in a regression, people find it difficult to communicate with me because they are so relaxed. They are experiencing emotions and visions or memories, but find it difficult to physically speak of them. Sometimes, they will wait until after the session and then tell me all about it.

Sometimes people also ask me if a past life memory could not actually be a dream. It is not and the difference is quite clear. For one thing in a dream you are unaware that you are dreaming and are caught up in the scene. Also in the dream, you are almost always yourself. You may be witnessing something strange and unfamiliar around you, but you are still your present body and personality. Also, dreams are sporadic and do not follow linear life-like patterns. One minute you are talking to your father who suddenly changes to your sister, etc. Dreams jump about continually.

Past life regressions, on the other hand, do follow linear life-like patterns. You do not jump about in a regression and people do not change into other people. A past life regression will move from beginning to end, although you are able to skip time and move forward and backward if the regression therapist asks you to do so.

A past life regression also makes sense, unlike a dream. It unfolds like a natural life and the interesting part of it is that while you are in the regression, you do not usually see the psychological patterns of the life or the personality. Why? Because you are in it, rather than outside of it.

Just as in real life, it is difficult to see our own patterns until someone tells us about them. As well, in a regression, you are not your present self, but someone else. You feel the body you are in and you feel the different personality you are in.

One of the most important reality checks is the emotions of the lifetime. It amazes people how they can be having a wonderful day and then suddenly, during the regression, they are overcome with emotions from a previous life.

The interesting thing that also happens during a regression is the split personality. For instance, when I experienced myself in my first regression as Catherine Graham, I found myself crying hysterically at the death of my father, who had just burned to death in a fire. I was screaming and sobbing, yet, at the same time, the present day Laurel, which was still a part of the experience, was judging the whole thing.

In other words, you maintain an awareness of being both your present day self and the person in the past life. The present day self often has a difficult time understanding why you are so emotional over some stranger.

The present day self is the logical self which is always there. This logical self often finds it disturbing if you start to become emotional in a regression and tries to judge you for it. For instance, in my regression into Catherine Graham when I was sobbing uncontrollably, my logical self was telling me to stop blubbering and making a fool of myself in front of the hypnosis therapist.

My logical mind was telling me that I was an idiot to be crying over this little man with a beard. That he couldn't possibly be my father. My father was six foot three and didn't look at all like this small little chubby faced man.

However, even though the logical mind tries to disengage you from the emotions by convincing you that you're making a fool of yourself, you still stay in the regression and in the experience. Why? Because it's an important part of your healing and this emotional past life has come up into your conscious memory for a reason. That reason is usually to heal something that is unresolved from the past.

Which is, after all, the point of having a regression in the first place.

CHAPTER NINETEEN

How To Be A Regression Therapist

THE REGRESSION TECHNIQUE IS BOTH simple and easy. It is a relaxation of the body in order to allow the brain waves to slow down. This is actually a form of self-hypnosis as the person you are relaxing is focussing on the various parts of their body. The regression therapist is simply telling them which part of the body to focus on and how to move deeper within.

The client is always in complete control and can open their eyes at any time. The client is not the victim of the regressionist. The regressionist is simply telling the client where to focus their awareness, but the client is the one who has to do it.

A regression therapist also cannot make someone have a past life memory, the client has to allow it to happen, by allowing themselves to relax and by opening their mind to receive the memories.

The regression therapist is actually acting as a guide and helps the client to move through the lifetime by asking them questions.

When I teach workshops on how to become a past life regression therapist, I often tell people that it takes a number of things to become a good therapist.

1. You need to be caring and compassionate;
2. You need to be able to soften your voice and be patient;
3. You need to heal your own past life emotions first; and
4. You need to be nosy.

Nosy? Yes, nosy. The best regression therapist needs to continually ask questions about the client's experience. That means continually asking - "what's happening", or "what are you experiencing now."

When a person is in a regression they are relaxed and distant from the present and often they are reluctant to tell the therapist the details about what they are feeling and experiencing. This is why the regression therapist needs to be inquisitive and continually ask them to share the details.

I often joke in my workshops about how a regression therapist will spend most of the session saying, "What's happening next?" and little else.

Once the person is in a regression, there is little for the therapist to do except to encourage the client to share what they are experiencing, and this means being nosy.

If you are choosing to become a regression therapist, or even to help friends and family to better their lives by releasing previous past life blocks, it is important that you cleanse your own issues first. The reason for this is that if you are helping someone move through a previous life memory in regression and they begin to remember a traumatic event, they will usually become emotional. If you have not released your own emotional baggage from the past, and that includes this present life as well, then you will find yourself becoming triggered by your client's emotional outburst and you will become emotional and unable to be helpful and encouraging to your client.

Inevitably when I teach a workshop someone will begin to release some emotional pain from the past and sure enough, those that are sitting around and watching start to cry as well. They are being triggered by the person's emotional pain because they still have their own pain within themselves.

Once you have moved out all of the old emotional energy from your previous lives as well as the present life, you will be able to be a much better regressionist, as you will be able to encourage someone else's emotional release, rather than be triggered by it or even afraid of it.

I have heard of many instances whereby a client was beginning to release an emotional trauma when their therapist began to calm them down. Often the therapist believes this is in the best interest of the client, but it isn't. It simply causes the client to push back down the emotions that need to surface and be released.

Most therapists are able to deal with simple emotional pain being released in the form of tears and/or gentle sobbing. But when a client begins to show signs of hyperventilation and/or locked jaw and uncontrollable teeth chattering, most therapists become helpless and find themselves trying to calm the client.

This is not healthy as the old energy which the client has been holding onto for untold lives is finally surfacing and needs encouragement to be released.

If a client does not feel safe and encouraged to move into their deepest pain and emotion, they will not allow it to surface and/or they will push it back down if it tries to surface.

This is why a good therapist is one who is able to not only be around intense emotional pain, but who can encourage the client to move into it fully and to express it fully.

This often means encouraging the client to yell and scream at the top of their lungs, something most people do not enjoy being around.

When I begin a workshop teaching people to become past life therapists, it never fails that everyone at the beginning wants to become a regression therapist. At the end of the workshop of say eight to ten people, usually only one will decide that they want to.

The reason is simple, most people find it very difficult to be around those who are expressing intense emotions.

However, if you, the therapist, first release your emotional baggage from the past, you will find that you are not triggered at all by people's emotional trauma. In fact, the opposite is true. You will find yourself encouraged by it and amazed at the intensity of pain that people hold within their bodies and energy fields for so long.

A good regression therapist sees the emotional release as wonderful and powerful as well as freeing, and is fully willing to encourage the client to express themselves as loudly or intensely as they possibly can.

A good regression therapist will also try to encourage the person to release their emotions by expressing sounds and often yells or even screams, with the client.

The reason for this is that when the client realizes that you, the therapist, are going to express sounds and or yells with them, then they feel safer to do so.

I will explain more of how to release energy and emotional trauma in the next section.

A regression therapist also needs to create an environment of safety and comfort for their client.

Often during my years of individual regression therapy, people would comment on how safe and comfortable they felt when entering my home, which is where I worked. I created a space with soft warm colors and a spiritual atmosphere, with aromatherapy essences, flowers, a few large crystals and some candles in the rooms.

In the actual regression room, I created a simple twin bed in a lavender colored room with a chair for myself and a table with flowers as well as a stereo. There was little need for anything else.

The reaction I received from people when entering my space was extremely positive. Often people spoke to me about having been to therapists such as psychologists, etc. and found themselves in a clinical environment with little to comfort them and so they found it difficult to relax and feel safe.

By creating a warm, homey environment, you are inviting people to feel relaxed and welcome.

It is also very important to comfort people when first meeting them as they are most often anxious about the experience for the first time.

I would always have people come into my living room and sit in a comfortable pink love seat with big pillows as I sat across from them. Then I would explain to them how regression works and I would ask them about their present lives and if there were any problems that they would like help with.

It is very important to take approximately half an hour when first meeting with a new client in order to get to know them and in order that they get to know you and become comfortable with you.

If a person feels safe with you as their regression therapist, they are more willing to relax faster and to allow their most emotional memories to surface immediately.

I often spoke with people who had been to a clinical psychologist or hypnotist who regressed them into a past life where little happened. If they did have a memory surface, it was usually a simple, boring lifetime, which seemed to have little effect on them and they certainly didn't release any emotional pain from the past.

The reason is simple, they didn't feel safe enough or comfortable enough with the psychologist or hypnotist to allow the most traumatic memories to surface.

There needs to be a level of trust between the therapist and the client in order for a profound experience to surface. This is why it is important to spend some time getting to know your client before you regress them.

Being a good regression therapist also means not being afraid to offer support and compassion.

I often explain in my workshops that a good therapist is like a good mother, you need to be loving and compassionate and not afraid to show it.

So often in our modern society filled with theories created by the psychology profession, we are taught that it is not right to touch someone. That we must only offer comfort with words and not with touch. I do not agree at all.

When you are experiencing an emotional pain of some kind would you rather have someone talk to you about how they understand your pain and are there for you, or would you rather be held in their arms.

A touch can mean so much to a person who is in an emotional trauma.

Years ago I found myself taking a course with hundreds of other people on inner child healing. The people were positioned in circles of ten in a huge room with about one hundred people, all sitting on the floor on pillows.

Then we were encouraged to close our eyes and move into our childhood issues whereby after a while some people would inevitably begin to bring up some emotions.

I was then greatly disheartened by the experience as I began to instinctively move towards a person nearby who was in distress to be supportive.

During my experiences with inner child healing and regression, I found it extremely helpful to simply get behind a person's back and gently hold them from behind. This encourages the person to lean back into your body and to really release a lot of emotional pain.

During this workshop, however, I was immediately told to stay put and to allow the person to release their pain, alone. No one helped them except to say a few words of encouragement, which did nothing.

I saw something then that I will never forget. The man who had begun to cry suddenly stopped crying. He had once again stuffed his emotions deep inside. Why? Because no one was helping him to release them.

In our society it is especially hard for a man to release old emotions and I truly believe that they need extra encouragement and loving support in order to do so.

A few moments later into the workshop, a woman near me began to feel an emotional upsurge within her and she began to sob. At that point a so-called assistant quickly helped her up and ushered her out of the room.

Their reason for this, as I learned later, was to ensure that others in the group were not disturbed. However, when a person is experiencing an emotional trauma, especially an inner child traumatic memory, I believe it is wrong to usher them out of the group. This creates a feeling of banishment and shame and signals to the subconscious that when one expresses themselves, one is ostracized. It is a negative signal to the subconscious and soon the person will stuff those emotions back down again as they have been given a clear signal that it is not safe or appropriate to express themselves within the group.

During my first experiences with workshops I learned some valuable lessons about comforting people.

One workshop had been about a natural energy form of healing called Reiki and it was being given by a woman who had a doctorate and many years' experience as a Reiki teacher.

As I was relatively new to the subject, I was intent on learning and watching. I had little understanding of natural energy healing methods and reacted on instinct when one of the women in the group who was lying in the center of the circle of us others, began to feel an emotional upsurge.

We as students were then encouraged to place our hands on her body in a flat position which is taught as the Reiki hand positions. The woman on the floor was sputtering and trying to control her emotions as the Reiki teacher encouraged her, with words, to express herself.

It was obvious to me that the woman did not want to embarrass herself in front of strangers and was trying to express her emotions in a gentle and safe manner.

I watched and followed instructions as the group continued to lay our palms on the various parts of the woman's body. After approximately fifteen minutes of this the woman had successfully stuffed her emotions back down and was calm again.

Then the Reiki teacher instructed her to sit up and pronounced that she was now much better and looked like a new being again. Naturally, as students not knowing any better, we all agreed. Although, I couldn't help but feel that something wasn't finished yet. I could immediately sense that the woman had not, in fact, released anything yet, and had only succeeded in stuffing her emotions back down.

The woman then stood up and the teacher announced how wonderful the whole experience had been and now we should all take a tea break after that intense experience.

I naturally thought to myself, if that was intense, then these people have never truly expressed a serious emotion in their lives.

I then gravitated to the woman who had just undergone the "intense" experience and I noticed she was shaking slightly and she seemed tense. I moved behind her and simply wrapped my arms around her and laid my cheek against her ear.

Suddenly the woman leaned back into me and began to sob uncontrollably. The sobs became deep, wracking sobs and I helped her down to the floor to a sitting position and kept myself behind her. I encouraged her to lay back into my chest and she moved into an even deeper emotional outburst. She then began to scream and shout that she was being burned to death.

Soon everyone came around and began to lay their hands on the woman in the Reiki manner while the teacher watched from the side and encouraged people to place their hands on the woman. I then instinctively began to breathe heavily with the woman so that my body moved in rhythm with hers and I whispered in her ear that I would go through the pain with her and that I wouldn't let her go. She immediately began to yell out loud as she recalled her past life memories of being tortured to death.

The others in the room also became triggered by the experience and began to cry as well and in a matter of minutes, everyone in the room had bonded to each other from their hearts.

After a while the woman became deeply relaxed and calm as well as exhausted. She had released an immense amount of energy and wanted to sleep.

An amazing thing then began to happen in the workshop. Whenever someone was placed in the center of the circle of people, they wanted me to be at their head and soon they were gravitating to me for support and love.

After the workshop, the teacher took me out for dinner and commented with much concern, that she had lost the workshop to me. We discussed it, as we were friends, and tried to figure out why that had happened. We realized that the people needed more than just a laying on of hands when emotions began to surface, they needed holding and a feeling of safety that someone was actually going through it with them, by breathing with them and even yelling with them, which I did as well.

By making the same sounds as the person releasing the emotion, you will encourage them to make a bigger sound, thereby intensifying the release of energy and healing faster.

During my next workshop and the ones following, I began to follow my instinct more and more and positioned myself behind someone when they began to feel emotions rising. I would simply hold them from behind their back and this simple act would encourage them to feel safe and loved enough to release with ease.

I realize that the modern methods of psychological practice is to respect boundaries. But offering love in my opinion is not stepping on someone's boundary, it is comforting and healing. Every person that I have helped in my years of work have expressed how much it helped them to release when I held them.

In our world of boundaries we are often rarely held and comforted anymore and certainly we are even more rarely held from behind our backs. We may hug each other from the front, but not from behind.

To be held from behind is quite a different feeling. It is a feeling of support and safety. Our backs are always open and rarely do we feel the tremendous safe and comforting love that is transmitted through the back when we are held that way.

Being held from the back encourages us to relax into someone who feels stronger than us. It gives us a signal that we are being cared for by a strong being. Being held from the front does not give us this feeling of support.

I highly recommend when you want to help someone feel loved and supportive, hug them from the back and allow them to lean into you. This will have a tremendous effect on them and it takes very little on your part to do it. Becoming a good therapist means not being afraid to love people and to show your compassion for their suffering. Words alone are, in my opinion, not an adequate expression of compassionate support and encouragement.

I have had numerous therapists which I have trained over the years tell me that they had come across a difficult regression whereby the person was unable to see much visually but was, in fact, feeling fearful or anxious and when they, the therapist, touched them gently on the belly or even head, the person immediately began to release the emotions they were trying to control.

We as a society in general are very controlling and have been taught that it is inappropriate to express emotions around others. So it's natural that a person is going to be resistant to sudden outbursts of cries and/or screams. They will almost always need encouragement from the therapist that it is safe to do so and they will not be judged for it.

CHAPTER TWENTY

Releasing Energy And Trauma

As I have stated earlier in this book, we are all energy vibrating and pulsating through our cells. This is our source. We carry our energy from life to life. We are also not one set amount of energy. We increase and decrease the energy which we hold in our bodies which we use to attach to emotion.

When we experience a trauma, we are increasing our energy and attaching an emotion to that new energy. Energy itself is not emotional, but with our personalities and egos, we attach emotions to energy. So to release energy, we do not necessarily need to release it exactly as it was created.

In other words, if we create an angry emotional energy through a situation with someone, we can, in fact, release that angry energy in two ways. One is by expressing it in an angry manner which is the most common way and most people believe, the only way. Or, we can express the anger in a healthy way, by deep, rapid breathing and emission of loud vocal sounds and rapid body movements.

We use past life regression and present life regression to awaken memories of previous events when we created an emotional energy which has not, as yet, been released. We carry these emotionally charged energies like little bombs within our bodies where they sit and disrupt our present lives, always looking for ways to erupt and be released.

This is how past events, which seem to have no basis in our present lives, affect us and cause present day difficulties.

For instance, an anger or fear created in a past life has an actual energy formation which is lingering within us and looking for an avenue to be released.

So we go through our lives creating triggers and problems which are, in fact, related to that past event and have little to do with our present life.

The purpose of past life regression is to remember the event which created the emotional energy and then to release it through emotional expression and deep breath work. This happens often in family relationships. We first need to realize that we reincarnate with the same spiritual energy beings over and over again in order to learn and evolve by experiencing situations together and by then balancing them in future lives.

A perfect example of how energy carries and affects our present is the situation of Janet. Janet had grown up in a family of four. All of the children seemed to get along fine with the parents but for some reason, Janet and her father had a very fiery relationship, filled with angry outbursts and a desire, on Janet's father's part, to be verbally cruel to her. Her father did not, however, react the same way with the other children, only to Janet. He would always put her down and try to sabotage anything she did with her life.

Upon doing a regression, Janet found herself in a previous life where she had been an overprotective mother to a young girl named Suzette in nineteenth century France. She did not realize in the life, however, that she was actually stifling Suzette's creativity as an artist and found herself continually criticizing Suzette. Suzette eventually began to withdraw into herself and rarely spoke to her mother, who did not understand what the problem was.

Suzette had, in fact, created a bitter and angry emotional energy and was holding it inside of herself as she had no outlet to release it and she seemed afraid of her mother.

After looking carefully at the life and then moving through Janet's previous life death experience and into the Bardo state, Janet realized that she had, in fact, been quite cruel to Suzette, without realizing it during the life itself.

She also discovered in the Bardo state that Suzette was now her present day father. A father who was carrying forward an angry and bitter emotional energy towards Janet.

The trick now was to heal that experience, when it was in fact, her father who was holding onto the energy.

This leads me to a fascinating part of regression therapy.

When there are two people involved in a past life regression whereby one is holding onto the energy, it can be healed or released by one of the people alone. In Janet's case it was possible for her to help her father to release the energy.

Most would think then that she would have to get her father to come and have a regression in order for him to release it but that's not the case. The reason being is that in a situation like Janet's there is an actual energy attachment between the two beings and if one releases it then the other is affected as well.

In Janet's case I had her create a situation of healing and forgiveness in the Bardo state. During this level of in between life awareness you are able to invite the higher self energy of those which you have experienced events with in the past.

I asked Janet to invite the higher self of Suzette to come and be a part of her experience. She then sensed and vaguely saw an image of light within her mind. This image then projected into Janet's mind that it was, indeed, the higher self of Suzette and Janet's father, who was the same being.

I then asked Janet to ask the higher self image if there was anything it wanted to say to Janet.

Immediately the spiritual image began to tell Janet how it had felt as Suzette and how Janet had been wrong to be cruel and controlling.

Janet listened and told me what she was receiving which was a long barrage of feelings from the higher self of Suzette. I then asked Janet to convey to the spirit her side of the story, which included her realization that she was quite unaware at the time of the life of her cruelty towards her daughter. She explained to the higher self image that she thought she was protecting her daughter from undo rejection and harm in a man's world by sheltering her and eliminating her hopes of artist success.

I then asked Janet to ask the higher self of Suzette and her father for forgiveness for all she had done. The higher self responded with acceptance. Then Janet realized that there was a chain-like image of orange light joining the higher self with her own body. It seemed to be attached to Janet's belly area.

This is a common occurrence, as I explained earlier that energies attach themselves to other energies when there is a conflict that is still to be balanced.

I asked Janet to feel as though she were pulling out that chain of energy and giving it back to Suzette's higher self. She followed my instructions and immediately felt both a sense of relief but also a feeling of a hole of sorts in her belly area.

I then instructed Janet to breathe slow and deeply into the area where she had pulled out the energy and I placed my hand on the area so that she was better able to focus upon it.

Also, by me placing my hand on the area I was able to help her to strengthen the area with the natural emission of my own energy through my hand.

We all naturally emit energy from our bodies and it is always helpful in regressions to strengthen someone by placing a hand on the area that is weak.

After the regression Janet expressed to me her understanding now of why her father reacted to her as he did and she told me that she would try to be more patient with him.

However, I explained to her that her father would actually be affected by this experience as well because his higher self had been a part of the regression.

Janet naturally found it hard to believe that her father would actually ever change but she remained hopeful.

About three weeks later Janet telephoned me with excitement in her voice. She explained how her father had suddenly taken up running and for some reason, he no longer seemed to be behaving cruelly towards her. Even her sister had noticed how her father was no longer putting her down and had even encouraged her on a new development in her life.

She was curious how this had happened and I explained to her that his higher self had caused him to release the emotional energy through running and that because his higher self had forgiven Janet, there was no longer any reason for the father to hold onto the energy.

This may seem amazing, but it is more than an unusual occurrence. It is quite common in regression.

I will give you the example of Jim, a man of fifty who came to me to find understanding about his relationship with his brother, whom he had not spoken with in twenty-five years.

Jim could not really remember the cause of the split with his brother, but he remembered there was a lot of anger and bitterness and he felt unwilling to try to actually do anything about the situation.

He came to me not to experience a past life but to use regression to go back twenty-five years to find the cause of the split, as he could not remember.

As I normally direct the subconscious to find the root of the problem, Jim was certainly surprised to find himself in Russia in the year 1911.

He did not try to resist the regression as I had explained to him before we began that the subconscious memory banks do not know the limits of time and would take him back to the original cause of the problem.

In Russia he found himself a teenage boy of seventeen who had joined the army with his friend, who was called Gregorovich. His own name had been Ivan.

The two had excitedly joined the army and found themselves in the middle of a plot which they had no understanding. Ivan had been tricked into taking some documents to an officer which turned out to be a plot to incriminate someone, although Ivan did not know whom.

It turned out that Ivan's friend Gregorovich was then implicated in a murder which he did not commit and for which he was framed by an officer. The whole scandal seemed most confusing and neither Ivan nor Gregorovich really understood what was happening nor who was responsible.

What did come out of it, however, was that when imprisoned, Gregorovich heard that his friend Ivan had been the one responsible for the incriminating documents.

Once I took Jim, or Ivan as he was called, through his death and into the Bardo state, he was then able to look back through the life from his higher self's perspective and he received a greater understanding of what had actually happened by bringing forward the higher self of Gregorovich.

It seemed that Gregorovich had been set up to take the fall for a murder committed by his officer. Documents containing evidence for the false accusations against Gregorovich were given to Ivan to take to an officer in charge who then reported them. This caused Gregorovich to be imprisoned, where he soon died of cold and starvation. During his time in prison though, he continually thought about his friend, whom he felt had betrayed him. He died without being able to express his betrayal to his friend as they never saw each other again. Ivan had been transferred to a far off place.

In the present, this betrayal manifested itself in a bitter situation between the two brothers who fought over something completely trivial.

As I moved Jim's awareness to his present life, he saw that the actual present life argument was actually over a television movie they had watched about Russian history.

In order to heal the situation, I had Jim, while in the Bardo state, ask his friend's higher self to join him. He then asked for forgiveness and also explained to the higher self that he had no understanding of what was in the documents he was carrying and that had he known, he certainly would not have delivered them but would have helped his friend. He also explained that he was immediately sent away, obviously to avoid the two of them meeting again.

After the session, Jim felt relieved and saddened that he had spent twenty- five years in his present life being mad at his brother for something that was created in his previous life. He told me he would definitely get in touch with his brother now and try to find a way to make peace.

The next day I received a telephone call from Jim. He was excited and stunned as he explained to me that when he awoke in the morning his brother, whom he had not spoken to for twenty-five years, had actually telephoned him and asked if they could meet and make peace.

He asked me how that could have happened and I explained how his brother's higher self had also helped his brother to release the old energy and he just happened to get to the telephone first.

The above two examples show how truly amazing energy is and how one person's healing and release of old energy actually affects the lives and energies of those around them.

Energy is most commonly held in our bellies which is why you feel nauseous when you are in a confrontational situation with someone or when you are upset.

The belly area is the center of power and it stretches from the naval up to the solar plexus.

When someone is holding old energy from a previous life or from the present life, it is usually centered in this area of the body and this is why the breath is so important in moving the energy out.

When someone is in a regression memory which is related to an energy being carried forward to the present, the body will give signs to the regressionist that energy is indeed blocked and needs to be released.

One of the various signals the body will give is locked jaw, where the person finds it increasingly difficult to speak as the mouth and jaw area become tighter.

This tightening of the jaw is signalling that something from the previous experience needs to be expressed verbally as the energy is locking in the mouth. As well, the client may experience discomfort in the throat area including tightness and pain and in extreme cases, uncontrollable teeth chattering.

When this occurs there is an immediate need to release the energy that is blocked in the throat and mouth area. The client needs to be encouraged to speak out the feelings that were not expressed during the initial incident in the previous life. However, because of the intense tightness in the throat and mouth area, it is often difficult for the client to do so and they will need encouragement from the regressionist.

This encouragement can come in the form of asking the client to open their mouths and to blow as hard as they can as though they are blowing a trumpet. At the same time it is necessary that they be told to breathe deeply and when they exhale to blow with all of the effort they can muster.

If this is difficult, it may be necessary for the regressionist to gently pull open the mouth of the client and lightly massage the area in order to begin the movement of locked energy. Then to encourage them to speak aloud anything they feel that they were unable to speak during the actual event.

It is most vital that the regressionist always pay attention to the body of the client as it will often give subtle signals that there is old energy within the body that needs to be released.

Uncontrollable teeth chattering can make it difficult for the client to speak aloud any words or emotions that have been repressed and it will take the efforts of the regressionist to insist that they breathe more deeply and blow out a loud sound through their mouth.

When someone has energy locked in their mouths and throats, I find it very helpful to make the blowing sounds with the client in order to encourage them. As they are in the middle of a past memory and wrapped in the emotion, it can be difficult for them to move past it and they are counting on the regression therapist to help them move it out.

It's also vital at this point that a person's breathing be watched carefully. Often when energy has been held from previous lives, it can be an overwhelming feeling when it begins to erupt and the person will try to control it or push it back down by holding the breath.

If you notice the person's breathing being shallow or held, place the palm of your hand on the person's stomach and lightly push down as you encourage them to breathe deeply.

Having a hand on the stomach reminds the person to connect with their breath.

We have all experienced times when in an emotional experience or when we are crying, that we tighten the stomach and chest and we breathe either very shallow or we hold our breath altogether until it becomes uncomfortable.

It is quite common that people will tighten their chests and hold their breath when they are in an emotional past life memory, however, it is important to know that they will only hold it for so long. They will breathe again.

Often in my workshops students have voiced concern that someone could hold their breath indefinitely and die. This doesn't happen as it will become so uncomfortable that the person will only be able to hold the breath for a short period of time.

It is similar to a child who is trying to hold their breath to show how angry or upset they are. They can only do it for so long before it becomes too uncomfortable.

However, in order to encourage the release of the energy within the person's body, it is wise to help them to breathe regularly and deeply, otherwise they will try to stuff the energy back down, which is what they are doing by controlling the breath.

When a person is in a traumatic or emotional memory, they will not usually realize that they are holding their breath either and so it is up to the regressionist to remind them not to hold it and to encourage them to breathe more deeply.

I reiterate the necessity in encouraging the client to breathe more deeply because it is a natural occurrence that the breathing become shallow and weak during a regression because of the relaxed state of the body and the slowness of the brain's oscillations. However, it is the only way to release old energy. The breath must become deep and rhythmic when the person is showing signs of emotional distress or the body is showing signs of locked energy.

Another way the body will show signs of locked energy is by the hands. The hands will slowly move from a relaxed position and become tense and often turn to fists or claws.

When this happens, the body is showing that there needs to be some form of physical expression in order to release the energy from within. Simply having the client verbalize any emotions that were not expressed is not enough when the hands or body become tense.

In order to release the energy which is building in the hands, there needs to be an intense movement of the hands themselves.

Normally in this instance, I would gently lift the person's hands, one and then the other, make a fist with them and tell the person to gently bounce them on the bed. Then I would encourage them to express anything that comes into their awareness that they had been unable to express in the previous life at the same time as they bounce their fists on the bed.

When the bouncing becomes rhythmic, which may take a minute, I would encourage the person to begin to breathe much more deeply and to begin to pound the fists on the bed with greater intensity.

Again, this will seem like a great effort to the client who is still in a relaxed state of being and so it will take much encouragement from the regressionist to insist that they push that old energy out with deep breathing and preferably sounds or blowing from the mouth as well as pounding of the fists.

As a regression therapist, I would always help the person to begin the process, as often, especially if it is their first experience in regression, they will have some resistance to pounding their fists as they feel they may lose control and become enraged.

It's important, however, that they do just that - lose control. If they continue to control the energy within them, then they will never be able to release it and it will continue to disrupt their lives.

When teaching a regression workshop, I have come to realize that it is often difficult for most people to encourage others to express themselves emotionally, but it is vital if you are to become a good regressionist.

It is important not to be afraid of energy or emotional outbursts. No one is being hurt, in fact the opposite is true, someone is being healed.

It is also important to be prepared for the amount of emotional energy that can be released in a regression.

The calmest and most gentle of persons can suddenly erupt into gut-wrenching screams and rage and the intensity of their body's release can be incredibly powerful.

This is why it is necessary before undertaking to regress someone that you create a space where they can release with freedom. I have always given my regressions in a house where no one could hear the yells and screams, although sometimes I was amazed that the police weren't called.

I recall one experience with Susan who had been through various methods of inner child healing and re-birthing and was no stranger to releasing energy.

When she found herself in a lifetime being tortured to death by her then husband, she freely allowed herself to express the emotions which she was not able to in that life.

I was amazed at the powerful force of energy which emitted from this petite woman as she yelled and screamed aloud. I was absolutely sure the police would be knocking on my door any second and was quite amazed when no one came. Susan had been yelling, "Stop killing me. You're hurting me. Stop it!"

Maybe it's a sign of how neighbors don't want to get involved or maybe my neighbors were simply used to yells and sobbing coming from my home.

The point is, however, that you need to create a space where people can freely emit their emotions and if you can't then you have to offer them an alternative. That alternative is a pillow with which they can scream into.

Often a pillow gives a person a feeling of greater freedom to express as they know they will not disturb anyone. As there is still a part of the present self awareness, there is often a reluctance to completely let go and move into the true emotional intensity of the moment. When a pillow is offered, this can give the person an opportunity to really emit without worry of disturbing others.

When someone begins to feel an emotional upsurge, no matter how small or large, there is an energy that is locked somewhere within the body and it needs to move upwards, not downwards. Some therapists believe that energy needs to be "grounded" but this is only going to cause it to be repressed again. The energy needs to be pushed upwards through deep breathing and blowing through the mouth and/or making sounds or expressing emotions through words.

Whether or not a person has a tight jaw or hands, it is the breath that still needs to activate the movement of energy. However, it is also important that they verbalize any emotions that they were unable to in the past.

An important note here is that they express their emotions to the actual person or people in the event and not to you, the regression therapist.

For instance, if you ask them what they need to say, they might tell you, "I'm angry with so and so." You then need to tell them to tell so and so that they are angry, not you. Always encouragement them to speak their emotions directly to those in the regression that they feel the emotion towards, not to you. They need to make a direct contact with the image of the person in the past and this will then affect that other person's higher self as well and not simply the client.

Trauma and emotional energy can come up in a regression both during the event and during the Bardo state. Although I have spoken of how important it is to do much of the healing in the Bardo state, it is necessary to release emotions whenever they arise and not to postpone an emotional awakening until the Bardo state.

If the emotions arise, as they often will, during an event in a previous life, then allow and encourage the person to express their feelings then, don't wait for later. Then during the Bardo state you can again ask them if there is anything left to be expressed that had not been previously.

It will be most common that emotions will arise during the past life itself, rather than in the Bardo state, because in the Bardo state you are usually detached from the body and it becomes less intense.

There is a greater mental understanding and clarity whilst in the Bardo state but less emotion than when in the past life body and personality itself.

Extraordinary things can happen to a person when old buried energy begins to emerge. It is almost like ooze or puss within their bellies and it can create a feeling of sickness within them.

It is fairly common when a person begins to release energy that they feel themselves becoming sick and or they start to cough. This is a good sign as it means the energy is moving quickly and there is a lot of it.

However, it is important not to keep the person lying in a flat position when they feel themselves becoming sick or when they begin to cough.

The therapist needs to immediately help the person to a sitting position by moving behind them. Tell them to keep their eyes closed and they will not come out of the regression, but they will be able then to release the energy.

The energy then needs to still be completely released and it is common for people to feel as though they are going to throw up, although they rarely will. They will, however, sometimes feel the need to spit and for this reason I have always kept a small clean towel beside the pillow just in case. Then express to them that it is perfectly fine for them to spit up or throw up if they feel like it.

Remember, as energy is moving up from the belly it can feel like old stagnant food that wants to be emitted. Coughing as well is quite common and should not by any means, be suppressed. Keep a glass of water for the person nearby before beginning the regression, in case they need it afterwards.

When someone is lying down and begins to feel a choking or coughing, immediately lift them to a sitting position and rub their backs gently up and down the spine. This will encourage the movement of energy. Remember also that they are dead weight and you must lift them alone as they will be unable to help you.

I have often noticed in teaching workshops on past life regression that the encouragement and release of intense energy and emotions can cause fear in those just beginning to be regression therapists. However, there is nothing to fear. The person is not going to die, they are simply releasing emotional energy.

It is important to watch their ability to release, however. For instance, if the person is over weight, then it is obvious that they can only release so much at one time as they will become exhausted.

The client, however, knows when they can do no more and will either tell you that they can't express anymore or they will simply slow down and stop.

As a regression therapist it is necessary to encourage them to express intensely and with effort, but do not go too far and push them beyond their capability.

This is why it is necessary to watch the body and the emotions of the person. When the emotions have finished expressing and the body is no longer tense, then the release is over. If there is still an intensity of emotion and the person has become exhausted from deep breathing and pounding their fists on the bed, then you need to have them verbalize until they have nothing more to say.

It can be necessary to help someone verbalize when they are trying to release as well. This is not considered leading as they are already experiencing a past life memory and are simply stuck at how to release their feelings.

If you have a situation whereby the person has been unjustly accused or abused in a previous life, it is pretty safe to say that they are going to be carrying some emotions around that experience and need to release some energy through verbalizing their feelings towards the person or people in the experience.

If you notice a tightness in the body or the emotions are erupting and the person seems to be having difficulty expressing themselves, then it is necessary to help them by asking them to say things to the person or people in the regression.

For instance, I would ask the client what they needed to say to the person in the past life. If they replied that they didn't know what to say. Then I would ask them how they feel about said person. If they replied, for instance, that they felt anger towards the person, then I would ask them to tell that person, "I am angry with you!"

Then I would continue to ask them if there were anything else they would like to say to that person and that this was their only chance so they might as well take it and say whatever they feel.

If the person then says something like, "I'm angry with you," in a very soft voice ask them to take a deeper breath and put a little more intensity in the statement as a weak statement is not going to create a release of energy. They need to put some strength into their statements and the regression therapist is the one who needs to encourage them to do so.

If a person is very relaxed and trying to express an angry emotion and they state their anger very weekly, I would encourage them myself by stating the sentence out loud for them, with more intensity. Then I would encourage them to say the statement again as I did, with power.

Emotions carried forward from previous lives often cause people to lose their power and they find it difficult to then assert themselves in a powerful way during a regression. Therefore, it is important that the regressionist assist them by verbalizing with them the statements that they are not able to say with strength. By having them repeat the statements with greater strength, it is wise to also tell them that they need to take their power back now and show the person that they will not be walked over again.

It is almost as though the regression therapist is acting as a cheerleader and supporter who is sitting beside them and cheering them on to be strong again.

This sort of encouragement comes with practice and experience, but don't hold back when someone is in need. Think of the person as a dear friend and you are trying to help them be powerful again and to speak their truth.

On a rare occasion, a client can experience hyperventilation and uncontrollable shaking as well as teeth chattering. This is simply showing that there is an incredible amount of energy trying to move out. It does not mean the person is going into shock and needs to be calmed down. It is not the same as shock.

I recall teaching a workshop when the person being regressed experienced the above with great intensity. Her body was shaking uncontrollably and her teeth chattering.

One of the students in the workshop was a trained paramedic and when he saw the person's body he looked startled and jumped up. I asked him where he was going and he replied that he was going to call an ambulance. He stated that the woman was going into shock and we needed an ambulance.

It took my strongest voice to insist that he sit down again and watch. He found it very difficult to believe me and he then informed me that we need to try to calm her down.

I looked him straight in the eye and said we would do no such thing, in fact, we were going to intensify her release and get this energy out.

Naturally, this went against every part of his medical training. I informed him that she was not experiencing shock and that she was not injured anywhere in her body. Her body was experiencing an intense energy surge.

I myself experienced this energy surge when releasing some repressed energy and emotion with regards to having been raped as a teenager. My body began to shake uncontrollably and my teeth were chattering. I was unable to control it so I decided to try to intensify it by expressing all the emotion I possible could, which included rage and sadness. I focussed on breathing as deeply as possible and within about fifteen minutes, the whole thing was over and I felt exhausted but wonderfully free and light.

The same thing happened with the woman in the workshop. I placed my hand on her belly and told her to keep focussing on breathing as deeply as she could. I massaged her mouth and encouraged her to try to blow and make simply aahhh sounds.

It was difficult for her but she felt safe as I comforted her and explained that this was wonderful that she was able to release such an intense amount of energy at one time and that we would not let anything happen to her.

Within a short time the energy moved out of her and she was relaxed and extremely peaceful. The paramedic on the other hand had difficulty understanding what had just taken place as his training had taught him that one should calm a person who is undergoing such a tremendous bodily surge.

This type of energy surge is rare, but it can happen and if it does, it is vital that the regression therapist not move into fear. If the regressionist shows fear then the client will try to suppress the energy and it will cause them to feel sick and they will go home feeling worse than when they came.

Certainly after a release of intense energy, it is natural to expect that the person is going to feel weak and even a little nauseous, especially if they are hungry.

This makes it very necessary to be careful to tend to their needs after a regression. It is never recommended to complete a regression and usher the person out of your house. They are still in your care and will often feel shaky and light-headed.

After a regression where there has been even a small amount of energy released, I would always give the person plenty of time to simply lie on the bed as we discussed how the previous life experience had effected their present life and various other things that we could gather from the experience.

I would also explain about the energy they released and how it was important that they take care of themselves in a gentle manner for the rest of the day.

I would recommend that they have some comforting food as soon as possible and not to undertake any mental stress or too much activity for the rest of the day.

Then before I would actually allow a person to rise from the bed I would usually rub their feet and their shins as well as their hands and fingers. This allows them to send some energy into their limbs. The reason for this is that a person undergoing a regression is usually lying on the bed for a period of one to two hours or even more. They have disconnected from their present bodies and it is helpful to stimulate the feet and hands to ground their energy into the present body.

Then I would have the person sit up, but not stand up right away. It is important to offer them some water or refreshment and then to slowly stand up whenever they feel ready. Do not rush anyone to stand up or they will become dizzy.

When the person has stood, I would recommend gently rubbing their spine up and down as this will help them to feel less light-headed. As well when they begin to walk it is important that they take some deep breaths.

A light-headed feeling is common and will often remain for the rest of the day. To assist the person in feeling more grounded, it is helpful that they walk outside and take some deep breaths of fresh air, especially if they are going to drive home. Always make sure a person is alert and grounded before you allow them to drive anywhere.

If you notice a person is feeling too spacey to drive, offer them something light to eat like a banana and a cup of tea. This will help them to regain their strength.

It is perfectly natural for a person to feel residual energy for a few days after a regression. Especially if it has been an intense regression where a lot of energy has been released.

Small amounts of energy will often linger in the belly, head and hands and can cause a person to feel nauseous and light-headed for a few days. Always let the person know of these effects before you send them home.

I would always recommend giving people some exercises to strengthen themselves after a regression if they are feeling light-headed or nauseous.

First it must be remembered that when a person releases any old energy they are going to feel weaker. They need to be told to eat soon after the regression and regularly for the next few days. Dieting is not wise after a regression. The body needs fuel to re-strengthen itself.

Often people feel lighter after a regression and this is simply because they have, in fact, released energy which was weighing them down. Sometimes they like this feeling of lightness and they forget that they still need to strengthen themselves. If they don't they will often find themselves having bruises on their arms and legs as they are not grounded and will often bump into things.

To help a person restore their energy if they are scattered or light-headed, recommend having their backs rubbed vigorously each day until they feel stronger, which will usually only take one to two days. Also it is helpful to sit on a hot water bottle in the morning and evening, or whenever one feels light-headed. This will activate the energy in your tail bone which will pull the energy from the head down into the body.

It can also be very helpful to give the feet a reflexology massage as well as deep massage in the legs and the back.

All of these exercises as well as deep breathing exercises regularly throughout the day will encourage the energy to strengthen quickly.

It is also very common for a person to want to sleep a lot after a regression for the first few days. This is part of the healing process and should be encouraged. Part of being a good regression therapist also means being available for a client even after the regression, should they need to talk. I always recommend telling the client that if they feel any concerns or simply want to discuss the regression, to feel free to call and talk.

CHAPTER TWENTY-ONE

Adoption

THE REGRESSION TECHNIQUE CAN BE also used to bring up memories from the present life as well as from the previous lives.

I have used it to help those who have been adopted and want to understand what happened after their birth as well as those who have issues which seem to relate to their present life birth experience or simply to heal inner child issues.

The memory banks which we tap into with regression can be accessed to heal any number of issues which are not always necessarily based in previous lives. This is why I always stress the importance of directing the person during the technique to go to the root of the problem, rather than to a past life.

Problems that people believe must have a basis in a past life can often be related to present day issues.

When working with someone who wants to find out about why they were put up for adoption it's best to first discuss with them the possibilities in order to decide if they are truly emotionally ready for any possibility.

The reason for this is that there can be many unusual circumstances that lead people to give their child up for adoption and people do not always prepare themselves for such possibilities. Most people assume that their mother was simply unable to care for them and so gave them up for adoption. It's not always that simple and I recommend a discussion before hand to ensure that the person is ready to deal with whatever they find.

My reason for writing this is because of one client I regressed in particular. I will call her Jenny to protect her actual name.

Jenny came to me in order to find out if she could remember anything about her birth experience as she had heard me discuss the issue on a radio show and how it was possible to find out what happened at birth because even though we're infants, our higher self always has the complete understanding and a higher view of the event and we can access the memories through the connection with our higher self in a regression, which happens in the Theta brain state.

After regressing Jenny to her pre-birth experience where she was simply a spirit in the Bardo state, I asked her to find her future mother.

She soon told me that she could see a very young woman who could be no more than about 15. The girl in fact, was milking a cow in a barn on a farm. The girl seemed unhappy and tired as Jenny watched her from a position above her which is natural as she was still in spirit form.

Within moments Jenny saw an older man enter the barn. When I asked her if she knew who the man was, she replied that he was the father of the young girl.

The older man seemed gruff and abusive to the young girl and slapped her across the face apparently for being too slow at milking the cows.

As Jenny watched the scene she became increasingly annoyed but not emotional. I asked her if she wanted to continue and she replied that she did.

Jenny next watched as the father of the young girl threw her on the floor and brutally raped his own daughter. Needless to say Jenny was horrified and found it difficult to tell me what she was seeing. Again I asked her if she wanted to continue and she said yes.

Next Jenny saw the young girl many months later and obviously very pregnant. The girl was packing some belongings and then quietly escaped the house in the middle of the night. She was walking a great distance and finally hitched a ride in a truck. She eventually arrived in a city and soon found her way to a hospital where she gave birth to Jenny.

During the birth Jenny felt herself being pulled into her mother's body and I instructed her that she had a choice to re-experience the birth or to stay in spirit form and view the whole thing from her higher self's perspective. She chose to view it from her higher self's perspective in order to get a better understanding of what happened.

If she were to choose going into the body and through the birth experience again, she would only remember it from the perspective of being an infant, and little would be understood as she would have little or no capacity to see.

However, by floating above, she saw two doctors surrounding her mother and her mother in tears as the doctors convinced her to sign an adoption form. The mother then never saw the child again and within a week, Jenny was adopted by a loving couple.

As Jenny was no longer connected to her mother, she was also no longer able to see what happened to her.

After the regression, Jenny naturally felt emotional and wept a great deal. It must have been very difficult for her to come to terms with the knowledge that she had been created out of an incestual rape and that she had no idea of what happened to her mother.

What Jenny was able to find out during the regression was the area where the farm was and what the farm looked like. As the event happened only 30 years earlier, there was still a possibility that she could find the farm and possibly trace her mother's life from there.

We discussed the possibility of her doing that although she seemed quite concerned that if she did, she would most probably run into her grandfather, who was also her father and she was not sure she was able to handle that experience.

I never heard from Jenny again so I have never found out if she actually did pursue finding her mother. Her other option to find her mother was through the hospital.

The emotions that Jenny then had to deal with were complex and I encouraged her to try to release her pain, which she said she would, but she first felt more of a pain for her mother than for herself.

I asked Jenny after the session if she would have rather not found out about the incident. She hesitated for a moment and then replied that she was glad she knew. She told me that it was better to know than to be in ignorance and at least now she knew that she wasn't given up for adoption because she wasn't loved.

She understood that there was no possible way her mother, a young teenage girl with an abusive father, could have taken care of a child. She also realized that it was a wise decision on her mother's part to give her up for adoption. That way her mother was trying to ensure that Jenny had a happy life and wasn't scarred by the whispers and stares of a small farming community who would certainly have judged both Jenny and her mother, not to mention having an abusive grandfather around.

Jenny felt a renewed sense of love and respect for her mother along with a sense of sadness and grief at what her mother had to endure.

Obviously a case like Jenny's is rare but it's an important example of what can arise out of regressing to our birth experiences to find out why we may have been given up for adoption. It also helps us to realize that regression should not be used for entertainment purposes but to genuinely help those in need.

CHAPTER TWENTY-TWO

Inner Child

INNER CHILD HEALING IS ALSO something that regression can be used to help with.

In recent years there have been many books written about the necessity to heal our inner child in order to create better, more fulfilled lives. Why stop at our childhood, why not go back and heal our past lives as well.

We carry emotional energies from our childhood and birth the same as we carry emotional energies from our previous lives and I find it quite fascinating how regression can assist to heal our childhood and birth issues as well as our past life issues.

We use the regression technique in the same manner, only directing the client to go to the root of their childhood pain or issue, rather than a previous life. Or simply go to the root of the problem.

Children often carry emotions because they feel it's unsafe to express them. Usually that's true. If they express their anger or truth to their parents or teachers, for instance, they will usually be punished, so they quickly learn to suppress their feelings.

These feelings then sit in the belly area and solar plexus until they eventually begin to disrupt our lives.

It's interesting how often people feel that by remembering a childhood problem and analyzing it, that they have healed it and it shouldn't bother them any more. Wrong. It still keeps on ticking, just like a bomb, because they have never released the energy which is feeding the emotion and until they do, the issue will continue to affect their lives.

An interesting case was my friend Jerry. He was brought up in a family of ten boys and had little love or affection. Birthdays were acknowledged by having a small present waiting on the fireplace mantle in the morning with a card. That was it.

As he grew he naturally justified the lack of affection and the hardships from both father and mother as the effects of having too large a family. It's fascinating how we justify our childhood pains and lacks. Obviously we do so as a survival method.

Jerry had an incredible natural gift as an artist and although he expressed this gift, he was never able to truly feel that he was brilliant or to create any real acknowledgements for his talent, because he didn't believe in himself.

Obviously he didn't believe in himself because he never received the acknowledgements necessary for a child to create a powerful sense of well being and self worth that is necessary, especially for an artist, to create success.

Jerry found his adult life filled with being a bartender and having superficial relationships with women who were less powerful than himself. He had little or no time for his art and soon he became increasingly depressed with his life.

I offered to help him better his life by doing a regression and simply seeing what came up, although I knew that there had to be some issues from his childhood that were causing him to sabotage his art career.

During the regression, he went into his childhood memories and recalled how little affection or encouragement there had been. I asked him to look at his parent's images within his mind as they had been when he was young and express his feelings towards them. It was most difficult for him as he kept rationalizing that they didn't know any better and because there were so many children, they just didn't have enough to go around.

It took some time, approximately an hour, but eventually I noticed Jerry's hands turning into fists and his breathing had become very tight and controlled. I asked him to move to a younger age and if I recall correctly, he felt he was five years old and suddenly the emotions began to erupt with a great fury.

I immediately lifted his head and squeezed myself behind him and cradled his head and upper chest in my lap. I began to rock him and this gentle loving expression allowed his inner child to truly feel safe enough to emote the feelings of anger, neglect and pain which he had buried for almost thirty years.

His emotions erupted with such fury that he screamed and sobbed for almost an hour. Afterwards he was truly renewed and lighter and within a few weeks, he created being invited to live with a group of artists in another country where he soon became known as "The Master". Within one year he was teaching and selling his works and creating masterpieces.

CHAPTER TWENTY-THREE

Sexual Abuse

ANOTHER ISSUE THAT CAN BE helped with the use of the regression technique is sexual abuse. I have used it a great many times to help people who had either forgotten old abuse events or for those who had been unable to release the pain of the abuse and continued to suffer.

One such case was Martin. He had been severely depressed for over five years and had become a hermit. He found it increasingly impossible to eat in front of anyone, including his wife, and he rarely went out of his house. He hadn't worked in years and was retreating more and more into an isolated, fear based lifestyle.

Martin had undergone professional counselling offered through a government agency medical program for five years but the counsellors found they had not been able to help him as he was increasingly focussed on suicide and depression.

The first time Martin came to me he was extremely thin and couldn't look me in the eyes. He drove eleven hours in order to come for a regression and he was desperate to find an answer to his problem.

Martin was very careful to shelter the front of his body with his arms, crossing them over his solar plexus. This is a common sign of a person protecting their power center and should be noted when trying to help people. This immediately gave me the signal that Martin had lost his power at some point and was now trying to protect what little he had left.

Protecting the body by crossing the arms in front of the solar plexus is a common occurrence with people who have been sexually abused or experienced a similar loss of power, usually through abuse of some sort.

In order to create a sense of trust with Martin, I encouraged him to tell me about himself which he was perfectly willing to do. I was quite impressed to learn that Martin had educated himself about depression and psychological illnesses to an extraordinary degree. He had read every book about psychology and told me how he had often caused his counsellors to be at a loss because he already knew all the answers.

Even so, he still had no answer for his problem. He told me that he felt black inside and black all around him. Even when he was in sunlight he felt only darkness around him. He told me that his difficulty had begun approximately five years earlier completely out of the blue and didn't seem to have any basis. Martin was in his early thirties when he came to me.

I told Martin that I would not necessarily regress him into a past life, although I assumed that was where the problem lay, but would simply suggest he go to the root of the problem.

Martin regressed easily into a relaxed state and soon felt himself as a young boy the age of four. He looked around and was happily playing outside of his house when his mother came out to tell him that she had to go out and would be taking him to the neighbors to be babysat.

Martin had regressed not into a previous life as was expected, but to his present life childhood.

Martin soon found himself at his neighbors being cared for by a large middle aged man and his wife. He told me that he felt uncomfortable around the man as he seemed to be gruff and cold.

Soon Martin began to tell me about his terrible experiences at the hands of this couple, wherein he was taken into the bedroom by the man and sexually abused. Then, to make matters worse, the wife of the man entered and rather than being horrified, she shamed Martin and dragged him to the bathroom and roughly washed him.

In shock and feeling nothing but numb, the four year old Martin then ran out of the house and made his way to a nearby dump. He found an old green coke bottle and he began to stare at it intently. He stared at the bottle so much he began to feel something unusual happen.

He told me how a black veil was beginning to erupt from inside of him and it was surrounding him. Then he felt as though he were actually entering the coke bottle itself.

After he felt himself enter the coke bottle something extraordinary happened. Martin suddenly found himself walking back home and into the kitchen, where he found his mother had just returned. He cheerfully asked her what was for dinner.

The young Martin had completely forgotten what had just happened to him.

Martin's case is important because it shows us what the mind is capable of in order to survive horrific emotional experiences.

Naturally at the age of four, Martin was unable to deal with the intense emotions of having just been sexually abused as well as shamed and he found that by staring into the coke bottle he could actually send his black feelings and memories into it and bottle them up, hopefully forever. Then he was able to get on with his life as though nothing had happened. Until he got older.

It's common for childhood events to be suppressed in order that we may survive, but these events are by no means gone, they are simply stuffed inside. This suppression can last for many years but usually seems to surface either in the thirties or forties.

I assume it's because the person is simply more able to deal with emotional trauma when they are matured.

In order to heal Martin's emotional pain, it was necessary to release the pain that was still buried inside of him. Remembering is not enough and does not create a release of the energy that had been stored in Martin's body. We needed to find a way to get that pain and energy out for good.

There are a number of ways to heal childhood abuse issues but I have found there are a few basics.

The first thing to remember is that trying to emit the emotions while in the memory itself is not usually possible. The reason being is that the person is a child and a child is afraid to show anger towards an adult as the adult is the one who abused them and may do so again if they become angry.

This is the same whether a person is remembering a past life childhood abuse or a present life childhood abuse. Whilst in the child-like state, they are unable to express themselves fully because they don't feel safe enough to do so. They are too small.

So what do we do to release the pain? We ask them to grow up to their present age.

While still in the regression, I asked Martin to feel himself ageing to his present age, which brought his brain waves back up to an alpha level.

The reason for doing this, is that in order to heal his emotions, Martin needed to create an image of communing with his inner child and his neighbor. As this would not be an actual memory, but a created image, it was necessary to activate his brain waves to an Alpha level.

This isn't necessary in a past life regression as we do the interaction with the higher self of people whom we have interacted with and we do it in the Bardo state, which is not actually in a past life any longer.

With a present life healing, we cannot go into the Bardo state as we haven't died yet, and so we must lift our awareness to an Alpha level and create an image to use in order to heal. This is only necessary with inner child work as we want to help the inner child feel safer by growing up.

I then asked Martin to bring the image of the small boy that he was beside him. This only took a moment and soon Martin the adult felt himself looking at Martin the young boy.

I asked Martin to tell the boy that he had come in order to help him and to protect him. I asked him then to tell the boy that he would never allow this to happen again and that he was going to take care of the neighbors himself so that nothing would happen to him again.

I then asked him to bring forward his memory of the neighbors again. He did. He again saw the male neighbor. I encouraged Martin the adult to then express his feelings towards this man as he was now taller and more equal to the man. I also told Martin that he could invite his higher self to be beside him for moral support if he didn't feel strong enough, as this man was quite large.

To my amazement Martin then began to yell and scream at this man and his face became deep red and his fists clenched. He then explained to me that he felt the need to hit the man and teach him a lesson.

I encouraged him to do anything he felt necessary to get out his pain. An incredible amount of rage came out of Martin such as which I have never seen released before or since. It was powerful and wonderful to watch this man heal himself by releasing all of his rage.

Martin explained to me after that he felt the need to kill the man in his mind, as though by killing him in the vision, he was eliminating the man from his own energy and body.

After all of his rage was spent, I then asked Martin to look at the small boy who was still beside him. He told me that the boy had a tremendous smile on his face as though he were looking at his hero. I then asked Martin to pick up the boy and cuddle him which he did. He told me that he felt a tremendous amount of love from the boy and he himself as the adult felt wonderfully powerful and exhilarated.

The inner child is a part of our personality which remains with us throughout our life. We can tap into the emotional states of these inner children by relaxing our brain waves just a little, into an Alpha wave, and remembering them as they, or we, were.

In order to remember a buried memory it is necessary to go into a Theta awareness but in order to work with your present life inner child and create a visual image which is not an actual memory in order to heal, it's necessary to activate the brain waves to an Alpha level. This is simply done by breathing a little more deeply and instructing the client to age themselves back to the present but to remain relaxed and heavy in feeling.

After Martin had completed the session he told me that he felt incredibly powerful and although he was shocked at the memory as he had no idea he had been sexually abused, he realized that it made perfect sense and wondered why he had never had any recall of the event whatsoever.

We discussed the event with the coke bottle and how it was actually used by the child in an ingenious way to bottle up the pain in order that he be able to continue with his life in a normal manner.

I explained to Martin that the healing was not complete, however, and that he still needed to heal his feelings of shame projected upon him by the female neighbor and that after that, he needed to continue his inner child work and establish a greater connection with him.

Martin returned again the following week and worked out his anger towards the female neighbor in the same manner and soon became an expert on inner child healing.

Within a month the change in Martin was extraordinary as both he and his wife then came to one of my workshops on past life regression healing.

It was the first time he had been able to be with other people as well as to eat with them during lunch.

Martin was an extraordinary case as well because he used his experiences to help others and within a year, both he and his wife moved to England

and opened a practice helping other victims of abuse as well as past life problems.

Martin came to see me about a year and a half later and I didn't recognize him as he had gained weight and looked so healthy.

I have worked with many cases of sexual abuse, both remembered and forgotten and I have found that the regression technique and releasing techniques work amazingly well and very quickly.

I have talked to numerous therapists over the years who have told me that it is impossible to heal childhood abuse issues quickly and that the client should expect to work on a weekly basis for at least a year. I think this is rubbish.

Regression does indeed work very quickly and I have seen it in practice. Another case in point is Anna, whose name I have changed to protect her.

Anna had perfect recall of her memories of childhood sexual abuse and had been in therapy for over twelve years. When she telephoned me she was curt and to the point. She asked me what my qualifications were and what I intended to do for her as she was tired of wasting time with therapists and psychologists who simply encouraged her to talk and talk until she was all talked out. She explained that she knew the problems and had expressed much anger over the years but her life was still messed up and she was incapable of having loving intimacy with her current boyfriend whom she was hoping to marry, but felt unable to.

When Anna first came to me I was astounded by her incredible beauty although she tried to hide it. She wore a moomoo type dress which hid her figure and she sat across from me with her arms folded across her chest in a protective manner. She also always crossed her legs tightly. She was assertive and tough in her manner and was making it quite clear that she knew everything about her psyche and wasn't going to waste her time with quack theories or practices.

I explained to Anna that I worked differently than a traditional therapist, as I believed that simply remembering the abuse was not enough. That she needed to release the rage that was connected with the incident, as well as heal the injustice of it, whilst in a theta or alpha level of the brain. In other words, in the subconscious.

I regressed her into the past just as I had with Martin and it was extremely painful for Anna to remember with such vivid recall the incidents of sexual abuse.

The difference with experiencing a regression and simply recalling the memory is that in the regression, Anna was actually feeling small again, whereas during previous therapy sessions over the years, she was recalling the memories through her adult mind. This avenue does not have the impact necessary to heal as it's easy to analyze and understand through the adult mind, but one has to go back into the child's mind and feelings in order to truly re-experience the moment.

This is the main difference with traditional therapy and regression therapy. I believe that in order to truly release the past, we need to not simply remember it, but to re-experience it, then we allow the flood of old energy to surface in order to be released.

In Anna's case it took a few months to work through all of her anger and pain as she had been abused a great many times from the age of four to twelve.

Again, the intensity of rage that came out from her was incredible and she, like Martin, felt the need to visually kill her abuser during the regression in order to completely release him from her energy and body.

Within a few months, Anna came to me and I was stunned at the sudden change in her. She was wearing skin tight leggings and a snug top, revealing a curvaceous and beautiful figure. She was beaming and laughing as she explained to me how she had just walked past a construction site whereby the workers, naturally, whistled at her.

She explained how, in the past, if she were whistled at she would become angry and aggressive, which is why she had begun wearing large loose clothes.

Now she sat on the couch with me in a lotus position, as she no longer felt the need to constantly keep her legs crossed. She felt great about her body and was ready for a sexual relationship. Interestingly, as Anna had come into her incredible power, she soon realized that her fiancé was no longer strong enough for her.

She had stayed with this man in the past because he was weak and non-assertive and of course, would never be a threat to her. Now she wanted a man who was equal to her increasing power.

Using the regression technique for inner child work is very fulfilling and beneficial although I recommend learning as much as possible about the inner child as it affects people's present lives in unusual ways, including manipulating events and causing illnesses.

The inner child is a part of our present personality and we are able to tap into that child by relaxation and simply inviting the child to come into our vision. Then it is as simple as asking the inner child how he or she is feeling and what they need.

CHAPTER TWENTY-FOUR

Eating Disorders

EATING DISORDERS ARE ANOTHER COMMON occurrence which can be helped by the regression technique. However, eating disorders are not usually created by past life emotional blocks. Rather, they are most often present life emotional blocks.

It is still possible, however, to use the technique in the same manner as you would a regression, but rather than directing the person with the eating disorder to a previous life affecting them the most, I would direct them during the technique to go to the root of their issue with eating.

To do this I recommend placing a few words on the door which is used in the regression technique in the time tunnel. Those words should be "eating disorder".

Whenever there is a specific issue to be resolved, I recommend placing the name of that very issue on the door in the time tunnel so that the subconscious knows exactly where to go and doesn't beat around the bush.

When I first underwent hypnosis to find the root of my insomnia I spent three months of weekly sessions trying to find the cause. If the therapist had directed my subconscious to go the issue of insomnia by giving a direct visual command, then I would have found the problem in the first session and saved a lot of money and time.

Instead, she simply relaxed me using hypnosis and allowed my subconscious to come up with whatever it wanted, which was a lot of clues to the problem, but nothing concrete because my mind wanted to avoid it.

The issue of eating disorders can have two causes. The first is that in a previous life one either starved to death or watched someone or many people starve to death whilst they indulged in food. This is quite obvious and by simply remembering the life and feeling either the sorrow of starvation and releasing any emotions around the issue, or by releasing any guilt about having food whilst others around us starved, we can heal quite easily.

An example of someone being affected by a previous life starvation is Elaine.

Elaine had found herself in a snow storm where she was unable to get out of the house for days. Four feet of snow had fallen and the whole community was forced to a stand still. However, it was Christmas and she had food in the house where she was staying although it suddenly didn't seem like enough.

Elaine's subconscious memory of a previous starvation was triggered and she began to panic and believe that she was going to starve, even though it was clear that it would only be a few days until the roads were clear and the house had enough food to last that few days.

The panic Elaine was experiencing was not logical and so gives us a clue that it was coming from a previous memory.

Many people carry on throughout their lives with phobias and fears that can easily be released if they would only look back into the past and find the true cause, then release the emotion around the previous event. Then they could get on with their lives in a much healthier and happier way.

Another case of a previous life starvation was Lisa. Lisa had the unusual habit of storing food in various places, just in case. Just in case what? She lived in a city and always had food nearby so I couldn't help but wonder why she felt the need to store food. She would always have a stash of chocolate bars in the trunk of her car, she said for "Emergencies".

In a North American city there is rarely an occurrence that calls for an emergency chocolate bar unless you are a diabetic, which she wasn't.

I asked Lisa if she would be willing to undergo a regression to find out if there were a previous life cause to her anxieties over starvation. She agreed.

During the regression she found herself in Russia during a winter storm. She was a female and had no food and was indeed, starving to death. She ended up falling into a snow bank and dying of the cold, although the reason for falling into the snow bank had been because of weakness due to starvation.

After releasing some of her emotions around the issue, which included, interestingly, anger towards her father in that life, who abandoned her, she was able to release the need to store food.

These previous life experiences with regards to starvation are easily healed and definitely are the basis for some eating disorders although it is much more common to have the cause for such disorders as bulimia and anorexia nervosa be in the present life, rather than the past.

I have had numerous successes with clients with the above disorders heal their lives by taking them back to the root of their difficulty.

Nearly every case I worked with had been extremely similar. Usually the female, as was most often the case, but not always, had experienced a loss of control at some point in her life.

Because of the loss of control, usually caused by someone such as a parent asserting too much control, the girl found that the only thing left in her life that she could control was her body.

There are innumerable causes to create a loss of control. Anything from abuse, either sexual, physical, or emotional, to a controlling parent who thinks they are doing the child good by pushing them.

I have witnessed clients tell me during regression about domineering parents who insist the child do various things with their lives, even if the child doesn't want to.

Insistence by parents often causes the child or adolescent to feel they no longer have choice or control over their lives or destiny.

They then begin a cycle of controlling their food intake and their bodies with the use of food. Interestingly, this usually annoys or upsets the parents who then try to control even more and the cycle worsens.

Someone with an eating disorder needs to go back to the first time they felt the loss of control. They need to remember the event and then heal it by using the inner child methods to release their emotions and to regain control by telling the parents, during regression, that they will not allow themselves and their inner child or adolescent to be dominated or controlled by anyone, anymore.

Then by learning to work with their inner child or adolescent and by building their own power again by telling others to stay out of their lives and learning to handle their own lives, they rebuild and learn to release such a tight control of their bodies.

Often with eating disorders as well as childhood abuse issues there are many incidents where the person felt control and choice was taken from them. Each of these incidents needs to be remembered and healed with both expression of bottled emotion as well as regaining power again by asserting one's voice to the offending controller.

The body is the last thing that a person has left to control when they feel stripped of their power and they will use it to show others that they will control their own lives and there is nothing anyone, including a parent, can do about it.

Every parent who has had a child knows that they feel powerless when their child has bulimia or anorexia nervosa and that is exactly the point their child wants to make. You may have been able to strip me of choice and control in other areas, but you have no control over what I do to my body.

Over the years, I have seen many young people heal their lives and their bodies by first releasing their frustrations at the controllers in their lives and then learning to regain their power, by making their own choices and not allowing others to interfere.

Choice must always be respected, even in our children. We should not have children simply to control and manipulate them. They are free and independent human beings and should be honored and empowered to choose for themselves. This creates strong and self reliant beings.

CHAPTER TWENTY-FIVE

Preparing For The Technique

THE REGRESSION TECHNIQUE IS BOTH easy to do and can be done by most anyone. However, being a good regressionist takes more than being able to read the technique. It means being able to help someone release energy and trauma as well as being compassionate and sensitive. It also means being able to help someone understand their previous life blocks and how they relate to the present.

The technique itself can be easily read but takes some practice, especially with the voice. I wish to emphasize the need to speak slowly when regressing someone and to blend the words together, not to speak in a stilted or stiff manner.

Interestingly, no matter how many times I state this in a workshop, people still speak in a stilted way and often far too loudly.

The voice is integral in regressing someone. If your voice is gruff and loud, it will be very difficult for the person to not only relax, but to drift deeper within to a Theta level.

What I always teach people to do when regressing someone is to relax themselves, that way the voice relaxes and becomes softer. Therefore, it's necessary to become very familiar with the regression technique before trying it out on someone. If you are unfamiliar with it, your voice will not be relaxed and it will not soften during the process either.

To begin the technique the voice can be quite normal but as you progress through the technique and are encouraging the client to relax and feel heavy, there needs to be a softening of the voice and an emphasis on certain words.

For instance, the word heavy. This word is used commonly throughout the regression technique and it is important to emphasis the "H" when saying the word. In other words take a breathe and say the word in a soft but heavy manner. This makes the word itself seem heavy to say and creates an effect of feeling heavy for the client.

Everything about the regression technique is about feeling and so to regress someone your voice needs to emphasis the feelings stated in the technique. Simply reading the technique in a monotone way with no emphasis on specific words will usually cause the client to fall asleep.

With regression we want to relax a person deeply but also keep them alert and awake.

When saying the technique it is also important to elongate certain words and/or blend them together without too much spacing in between. This way of speaking creates a continual flow of words which causes a person to relax whereas if the words are spoken in a very broken, individual way, the client will have a greater tendency to focus on the words rather than feeling what the words are telling them to feel.

In beginning a regression I always tell the person to feel what I am telling them to feel, for instance, to 'feel' their legs becoming heavier, rather than to focus on the words in their minds and analyze them.

Most people are analyzers and are not used to feeling their bodies relaxing and so they will go over the words again and again in their minds and not do what the words are telling them to do.

To get beyond this, it is helpful to emphasis the word 'feeling' when it says so in the technique. Also it is wise to stretch out the word 'feeling' in order to remind the person not to analyze it but to feel it. Say it as though it reads 'feeeeling'.

By stretching the words which suggest an action it helps the client to use their senses rather than their logical mind.

Other words can be spoken softly but usually without having to elongate them.

The key to becoming a good regressionist is learning to relax yourself as you are regressing someone. This will give you a sense of how to soften the voice.

Sometimes, if a person is having difficult speaking slowly and softly enough, I recommend they close their eyes and say some of the technique from memory. This way they are relaxing as well and their voice responds.

The relaxation and softening of your voice encourages the client to move more deeply and rapidly into a Theta state.

It must be remembered that someone being regressed for the first time is usually nervous and hearing the softness in your voice will make them feel more relaxed, even before you begin the technique.

I would always speak softly with people when about to do a regression as half the battle is already won if they are a little relaxed even before they lie down.

Lying down is important as well to having a good regression. My first regression was done in a sitting position and I remember finding it distracting as I had to hold my head up when it wanted to fall.

Having a person lie down on a bed is much more appropriate than having them sit in a chair. Then they do not need to be concerned with taking care of their present body. This allows their body to become heavier and more relaxed than if regressed in a chair.

A chair regression will usually only allow a person to relax to an Alpha level as they continue to be aware of their present body. This is why some people who have gone to have regressions in a psychologist's office in a chair, for instance, have not been successful.

In creating an appropriate space to do a regression, consider a place that is very quiet. As a person moves into an Alpha and Theta state their awareness becomes acute and they are more able to hear distant sounds, which can be very distracting.

Unplug any telephones and cover answer machines or turn the volume down. it is very disappointing when you are nearing a past life memory and suddenly a phone rings, which causes the person to come back to the present and you have to start all over again.

Next it is most important to be sure to empty the bladder before beginning a regression. The reason for this is that when the body relaxes, the bladder relaxes and it is inevitable that the client will suddenly have to pee in the middle of the regression.

Keeping the body warm during a regression is also necessary. As the regressionist you may feel that the room is quite warm, but the person being regressed will be quite a bit cooler than you. This is because they are slowing down the body's functions and energy and just like when you go to sleep, your body becomes cooler. Always lay a light blanket over a person's body unless it is a very hot day.

Music is often helpful during a regression, but usually only in the beginning. In choosing music, I would recommend a light instrumental assortment with no intense changes. In other words, gentle meditative type music. This music must be played very low as the client will again become acutely aware of sounds when they are relaxing and you don't want them to begin to focus on the instrumentation of the music.

It is important to be very quiet during the regression as well, especially during the relaxation technique as it is vital that the person be able to detach from the present situation and drift deeper within.

Because of this I have developed over the years a way of sitting completely still and even of sneezing silently. I realize this is not healthy but again, it can be very frustrating to be regressing someone and suddenly you sneeze and bring them right back to the present.

Always have something to drink beside you because it takes approximately fifteen minutes to move through the regression technique and often the throat will need to be lubricated.

Again this should be done silently. Do not clank your tea cup on a table or gulp loudly or especially do not sip loudly. Every move you make as the regressionist needs to be done as silently as possible. This is the most difficult thing for the regressionist to do.

This is also why I don't recommend having another person in the room watching. It is usually very difficult for people to sit absolutely still and not fidget or clear their voice or something of that sort.

Naturally as you become more familiar with the regression technique you will find yourself changing various words and sometimes shortening it a little, as some people are more relaxed than others and seem to move into the regression faster.

However, for first timers, I recommend sticking to the length of the technique as it is as you will not be able to gauge how quickly they are regressing and it is better to be too slow rather than too fast.

Throughout the technique I have placed in parentheses the word 'pause'. These pauses should be for at least three to four seconds. Words that I have underlined should have a greater emphasis as they are to create a feeling in the person.

You will be asking the person to create some visual images during the technique. This is possible as they are moving through the Alpha and are able to create an image. They will be able to create an image in the Theta only if you describe it completely, otherwise they are only able to receive images from their memory.

In time you will also find it necessary to change some of the technique more for your own benefit than the client's. The reason is that you will become bored with it and find yourself drifting and will forget where you left off. This is especially the case when you come to the part where you are counting the person down from ten to one which is done very slowly.

I recommend counting them down using your fingers to remind you where you are. This may seem childish but you will soon find you will forget which number you have just said because you are relaxed as well. I cannot count the number of times when I have forgotten which number I was on and I said the wrong one.

You must remember that the client is acutely aware and will definitely notice a change in the sequence of numbers and this will cause their logical mind to pull them back to analyzing, which causes them to accelerate their brain waves again.

As you are regressing someone you do not want to give their logical minds anything to use to accelerate the brains waves and you can bet that their logical self is looking for something to grab hold of. The reason for this is that the logical mind does not understand what is going on and will try to control it by pulling the person back to a Beta awareness.

I have heard amazing stories after a regression about how people's minds resisted the experience and how they tried to control and analyze throughout the technique.

This is why it is important to follow the technique and not to lose your place.

Also, if you decide in time to change the technique, be careful where you change it. During an Alpha and Theta brain state the person responds literally to what you say. In our everyday language we are not used to this and can be surprised when the person does not respond or responds in a different manner than expected to what we have said.

For instance if asking a person their name in a regression, I have heard people in my workshop ask, "Do you have a name?" The client then replies, "Yes". Nothing more. The regressionist then needs to ask, "What is your name?"

Over many years of testing various methods and techniques, I have found the following to be the best. It is simple and easy, which is important. You do not want to give the person large words which also causes the logical mind to begin analyzing. Keep everything simple.

During various places in the regression technique I have the words 'or option'. This is the area where you would insert certain commands. For instance, if you want to direct the person to a lifetime they may have led in China or a lifetime they may have lived in the dark ages, this is where you would insert that command.

Also if you want to use this technique for present life memories, then use this space where I have (or option) to tell the person, for example, that they are going back to their childhood or the age of four, etc.

Normally, I would simply state at that juncture that they are going back to either 'an important lifetime' or 'to the cause of their problem'.

For instance, if they have a block in their present life about worthiness, I would state, "You are moving back to the time when your block with your self worth was created." Or I could simply state, "You are moving back to the lifetime affecting you the most." This is the statement I would most commonly use.

When giving a person an image during the regression technique, such as imagining a tunnel or an elevator, remember to pause long enough so that they can create that image, approximately five seconds.

CHAPTER TWENTY-SIX

The Technique

TAKE A SLOW, DEEP BREATH and close your eyes. Tense your hands as tight as you can (pause) and relax them. Tense your legs and feet as tight as you can (pause) and relax them.

Now allow yourself to feel a sense of calm coming over you and a sense of peace as your breathing softens and your mind relaxes. (pause)

Bring your attention to the point between your eyebrows. Don't actually look there, just have your attention there.

Allow yourself to be in a pure black space as you begin breathing slowly and softly.

With every breath you inhale, you inhale a feeling of calm and peace. (pause) With every exhale, you exhale any tension and stress that you may be holding in your body. (pause) Breathing in and breathing out.

Continue to feel your breath becoming slower and more relaxed.

Now begin to feel your eyes. Feel as though they are becoming heavy in the sockets (pause). As though they want to sink deep inside of your head into a pure black space. (pause) Allowing your eyes to feel heavy in your head.

As your eyes become heavier, you allow yourself to drift deep inside your mind. Drifting away from all outside sounds. Just feeling your body relaxing and feeling your mind drifting into a pure black space inside your mind. (long pause)

You're going to become aware of your feet now. Feeling any tightness in your feet relaxing. The muscles are loosening and becoming soft. Feeling now as though your feet are becoming heavy. (pause)

Now feeling the calves of your legs and your knees. Feeling the muscles relaxing and becoming loose. (pause) Noticing your calves and knees becoming heavy. Heavier and heavier. (pause)

Feeling the tops of your legs now. Noticing any tightness beginning to soften now. As though all of the tension in your legs is pouring out of the back of them and causing your legs to feel heavier and heavier. (pause)

Becoming aware now of your stomach and abdomen. Noticing any tension being held there and allowing it to relax. Allowing the muscles to become soft and the whole abdomen and stomach area to become heavy and relaxed. (pause)

Feeling your breathing relaxing even more now. (pause) Once again you feel your eyes sinking deeper into your head as you move deeper within yourself. (pause)

You begin now to feel your back. Feeling as though all of the tightness in your spine and the back muscles are loosening and the tension is pouring out into the bed and floor below you. (pause) Your whole back area is becoming heavy and loose. (pause)

Becoming aware of your shoulders and the back of your neck now. Noticing any tightness and feeling it becoming loose and relaxed. (pause)

The back of your shoulders and neck are sinking into the bed and pillow, becoming heavier and heavier. (pause)

Feeling your arms and hands now. Allowing all of the muscles to become soft and loose. (pause) All of the tightness is letting go and your arms and hands are becoming heavy and still. (pause)

Feeling your chest area now. Noticing any tightness that you may be holding there and allowing it to relax. (pause) Feeling all of the tension floating away and your chest area becoming heavy. Heavier and heavier. (pause)

Becoming aware of the tightness in your head and face now. (pause) Allowing the muscles in your face to loosen and relax. Feeling your forehead relaxing, your eyes, (pause) your cheeks and nose, your mouth and jaw all relaxing and becoming loose. (pause)

Now your going to feel as though a warm wave of energy is moving through your body, starting at your head (pause) and moving through your body (pause) and down through your feet. Feeling it moving through you, relaxing you even more. (pause) Now one more wave of energy is going to move through you from your head through your toes. Allowing it to soothe you. (long pause)

You're going to feel now as though you're detaching from your body, beginning with your legs. Feeling as though your legs are detaching from you, as though they are no longer a part of you. (pause)

Feeling now as though your stomach and abdomen area are detaching from you. Easily feeling them detaching from your awareness for now. Letting them go. (pause)

Now feeling your torso from the neck down. Feeling as though it's separating from you. (pause) You're just a head now. Feeling as though you're just a head and now you're going to bring your awareness deeper into the center of your head. (pause)

Now feeling as though you're just a circle of energy, floating in a pure black space with no attachments to a body or personality. Just a pure circle of energy.

Your whole being is peaceful and relaxed but alert and in complete control. If at anytime you feel uncomfortable and want to discontinue, just let me know as you are in complete control.

Now I would like you to feel as though you're floating inside of an elevator. (pause) This elevator is about to move downwards, deep inside of the earth. As I count you down from 10 to 1 you're going to feel as though you are sinking deep down into the earth inside of this elevator. You will be able to feel the elevator sinking downwards as you move deeper within yourself.

Beginning now to feel the elevator moving down easily and very slowly.

10 - moving down inside the elevator, feeling it sinking down.

9 - relaxing as you feel your whole being sinking deeper into

the earth within the elevator.

8 - so peaceful and relaxed. Feeling yourself sinking downwards.

7 - sinking deeper within.

6 - moving down, deeper within the earth.

5 - so relaxed and heavy - heavier and heavier.

4 - gently sinking downwards - deeper and deeper.

3 - easily relaxing, easily feeling heavier.

2 - moving deeper down. Feeling the elevator sinking down.

1 - sinking down inside the earth.

The elevator stops sinking now and the doors of the elevator open and you find yourself floating into a long tunnel. (pause)

There's a light at the end of the tunnel and you find yourself drawn to move down this tunnel towards that light.

This is a time tunnel and you're going to start to float down this tunnel and back through time. You're floating back through time now and you may be aware of numbers moving backwards floating by you, like calendar pages turning backwards. (pause)

You're floating down this time tunnel and back through time. Back to a previous lifetime affecting you the most (or option).

As you float down this tunnel you're going to find yourself coming closer to the light. You notice that the light is beaming out from behind a very old looking wooden door. You begin to sense the door and see it more and more clearly now.

As you move closer to the door you're going to notice letters painted on it which read previous lives (or option).

Your mind knows now that you are moving back to a previous lifetime affecting you the most (or option) and you know in your being that you are ready to remember that lifetime (or option) that is affecting you. It is easy and perfectly safe to remember your past.

You're moving right up to the door now and you're going to notice it opening now and the light behind it beams out, beckoning you to enter and remember. (pause)

In a moment you're going to move through the open doorway and into the past life that is affecting you the most (or option). On the count of three you're going to float through the doorway and find yourself being pulled into a body in your past.

Feeling ready now to move through the doorway and into your past memories. 1 (pause) 2 (pause) and 3, moving through the doorway now (make a slight blowing sound). (pause) Being pulled into the body "Now" - (pause) and you are there.

IN THE BODY

ONCE YOU HAVE REGRESSED SOMEONE through the doorway and into the body you will come across a number of things which I wish to address before continuing.

First, each person experiences a regression in their own way. Some people have excellent inner vision which makes it easy for them to see absolutely everything with exquisite detail. I myself experience this detail with great clarity and have from the beginning. Not all people, however, have a strong inner vision and some may find it difficult to see much.

You may find that some people are more able to sense things rather than actually see them. Some people are also very auditory and olfactory, which means they hear and smell very profoundly.

This first part of the experience of connecting someone with the body and establishing vision or senses is the most difficult.

Because the person is not used to the experience they may find themselves denying what they are sensing or seeing because it is not as clear as they would have thought.

It should be explained prior to the regression that the inner vision is not like outer vision and it will not be as bright visually as say, a dream. It will usually be like a vivid memory whilst having your eyes closed.

Prior to the regression, I will suggest to the person to close their eyes and picture their present home and to describe the home to me. Then I tell them that that vision is their inner vision and the regression will be similar to that. Again, with some it will be more vivid than with others.

The first thing that needs to be done once you have taken someone through the doorway is to establish a connection with the body and to reawaken the senses. This is most necessary, because you have disconnected them from the present body and now you need to connect them with the previous body and its senses.

Some people will state how vague the visual is or how fuzzy. Sometimes the reason for this is simply that we did not have electric lighting in previous lives and often the rooms themselves were hazy and/or smoky.

Also it should be taken into account that we often experience having poor vision in our previous lives. Remember that eye-glasses are a fairly new invention. As well you may experience being blind in a previous life and so it's important to establish a connection with the other senses, such as smell, hearing and touch as well as the most important one, emotions.

It's also fairly common for a first time regressee to be a little controlling and resistant to moving into their previous life bodies and so there are a number of tricks we can use to encourage them to enter the memory and the body. These will be addressed in a later chapter.

Before continuing with the regression I would like to address some basic issues which are quite important. The main one is that the regressionist should never lead or place ideas into the person's experience.

This is a common occurrence with less experienced regressionists who are not confident enough to allow a person to have their own experience. They for some reason feel it necessary to enhance the person's experience by leading them with suggestive words into possible experiences that the regressionist feels should happen next.

Contrary to common belief, this does not work. I have practiced this theory during research sessions and experienced my subjects becoming irritated and annoyed that I would dare to suggest what they might be experiencing.

In other words, no one likes to be told what they are seeing or experiencing, so let the person have their own experience. There is no need for you to enhance it by interfering or leading.

Over the years I have come across many people who told me of their experiences with other hypnotists or regression therapists who continually made leading suggestions, which only caused the person to become angry and frustrated.

If you make a suggestion to a person such as, "Are you experiencing being angry with your mother now?" You will usually find yourself hearing a curt reply in return, "No, that's not what I'm experiencing."

The regressionst never needs to lead but to ask vague, non leading questions, such as, "What are you experiencing?" or "What are you feeling?"

If you want to ask a more specific question, then it is important to always give the person an option, so that you are not leading them. For instance, you may ask, "Are you a male or female?" or "Are you heavy, slim or in between?"

Always be sure with specific questions, that you give a number of options, then the person will not feel as though you are leading them and trying to control their experience.

A good regression therapist asks basic and simple questions and this is always enough. You want to pull the answers out of the person being regressed, not put the answers in, that will be of no use whatsoever.

During my workshops, I have often seen my students asking probing questions, which were often leading. It's a common mistake in a beginner regressionist, but one that must be corrected. Remember to pull the answers out of the person by giving them options and simply asking, "What's happening next?" or "What are you feeling?"

Also remember that it takes time to receive an answer during a regression. The vision needs to unfold first in the person's mind before they are able to tell the regressionist what they are seeing or sensing. So be patient.

CONTINUATION OF THE TECHNIQUE

ONCE THEY ARE THROUGH THE doorway and you have instructed them to be pulled into a body, continue as follows:

Now the first thing you're going to become aware of is your senses. Your sense of smell there is awakening. Your sense of hearing, touch and feeling and most of all your vision. (pause)

You're feeling as though you are looking down now towards your feet, it's getting brighter and clearer each moment - and your feet are there, they're becoming clearer and brighter, your vision is focusing on your feet. Colors and shapes are forming more and more each moment.

Very softly and with no effort, I would like you to tell me what you're noticing, if anything, that you're wearing on your feet. The first thing that comes to mind, don't judge it. (pause and wait for an answer).

Now moving your vision upwards, you're going to notice your legs now. It's getting clearer and more focussed. Noticing what you are wearing, if anything, and what your legs look and feel like. (pause)

What are you wearing on your legs?

Moving now even further up your body and noticing your torso. Noticing what you are wearing, if anything, and what your body looks like. (pause)

Tell me now what your body and clothes are like.

Now you're going to notice your hair, as though you are sensing it. What is your hair like? (pause)

Are you in a male or female body?

Can you tell me how old you are? The first thing that comes to mind.

Now you're expanding your vision outward. Noticing what's around you, it's getting clearer and brighter each moment. You're going to notice if your inside somewhere or outside somewhere. (pause)

What does it look like around you?

Is there anyone around you, or not?

What are you doing in this place?

What is your name, the first thing that comes to mind?

What country are you in, the first thing that comes to mind?

What year is it?

Let's go to your home now - you're arriving there now. (pause)

Noticing your home, what does it look like?

Do you live there alone or with anyone?

How do you feel emotionally now?

Try to find your mother now, (pause) - where is she?

What does she look like?

How do you feel about her?

Find your father now.

What does he look like?

How do you feel about him?

Let's move through your day. (pause)

What are you doing?

Are you happy or not?

Do you have any friends or people you love? - Find them and tell me about them.

Let's move now to an important time in your life - moving there now (pause). You're there.

Looking around you again, noticing where you are. (pause)

Where are you now?

How old are you now?

What is happening around you?

How are you feeling emotionally?

Spend some time now playing detective. Ask questions but do not lead them in any way. Keep asking what is happening next and how they're feeling.

If nothing seems to be happening, move them forward in time again by approximately five years, or suggest that they go to an important time in their life and suggest that they arrive there now.

You can easily move people back and forth through time in the regression simply by making the suggestion and giving them a few seconds to get there. It must be remembered, however, that you then need to encourage them to establish their visual senses again by suggesting that they look around and see where they are and see how old they are now and what they are doing.

Sometimes it is necessary to move people back a little further in time from where they have arrived.

For instance, if they have arrived at a point of being judged for something or are in prison, then you want to suggest that they go back in time to the point before they became imprisoned or judged, in order to find out what happened to get them to that point.

Often people will arrive in a regression memory during the most intense moments and it is necessary to take them back further in order that you get a complete understanding of what lead up to the events in the first place.

If you move someone forward in time and they find themselves unable to connect with a vision or they feel themselves floating, then they have gone beyond their death and you need to move them back again, preferably to the point in time just before their death. Then ask them what is happening and what happens next.

If the lifetime the person has entered is difficult for them to see or even sense, then it can often help to have them feel themselves lift out of the body and float above it, then look down and find their body and see what it is doing or where it is.

I have come across this a number of times when a person arrived in a memory where they were either buried alive, in a dungeon or perhaps even blind. By asking them to lift out of the body and float above it, then look down and see it, they were much more able to find out what was going on.

Also, if a person enters an experience in a previous life that seems unbearable to re-experience, I would recommend again having them lift out of the body and float above it, then look down and watch the experience. This is the memory from their higher self's point of view.

They will usually still be able to experience the emotions of the life, without the actual physical sensations being remembered with too much intensity.

Although physical sensations, such as burning or torture, can be re-experienced, it is a memory of the pain. However, because memories can be very vivid, it is common that the memory of pain or torture can be acute and it is not necessary that a person linger in such an experience.

The point of regression is to heal and learn from the memories of our past lives, not to re-experience suffering to remember pain.

Once in a while you will come across someone who does not want to lift from the experience of torture or suffering because they feel it is important to remember.

I always recommend asking a person if they feel the experience is too much to feel and ask if they want to lift from it, or not. Give the person the option to watch the scene from above their body if it seems too intense.

For instance, if the person is being physically tortured or burned at the stake, it is much easier to watch it from above. They often simply need to remember what happened enough so as to trigger any emotional energy which they have repressed, not to undergo the torture again.

Remember that past life memories are used to trigger emotional blocks and not to feed anyone's desires to listen to morbid or horrific events. It is not necessary for a person to linger in torment. What is more helpful is to find out, for instance, who judged the person and sentenced them to be tortured than the torture itself.

For instance, a torturous experience itself is not usually the cause of an emotional block, it is usually something such as the person having been wrongly accused or having been set up.

These are the things that need to be discovered in a regression. It is the emotional blocks that usually occur between people rather than the events that occur as a result of the exchange.

It is also important to remember that simple events in previous lives can often be the cause for emotional blocks.

Often I have heard of regression therapists moving people towards what they call the exciting or intense events in a person's life in order to create an intense experience. However, it should be noted that those intense events are often the result of a simple exchange, which is the actual cause of the event.

It is the cause that is the most important, not the result.

Focus on trying to find the cause to emotional blocks, rather than intense events in a person's previous lives.

It is also important to remember to ask a person how they are feeling throughout the regression. This can be a way to trigger the release of some blocked emotions. Also continue to watch their body signs, especially the hands, mouth and breathing.

If the breathing and/or hands become tight, then the emotions are trying to surface and you need to probe the person as to what they are feeling and what they need to express or say that they had been unable to.

After you have moved through the life and received all of the information necessary to understand it, then it is time to take them through their death and into the Bardo state.

THE BARDO STATE NOTES

WHEN YOU MOVE SOMEONE THROUGH their death experience it is important to reiterate that it is easy and simple and that they will simply float above their bodies.

It is helpful when having someone first leave their body that you allow them time to look down and see where they left the body and where they are being buried, if they are? This can also be helpful if a person chooses to later find their grave.

Whilst in the Bardo state many people will find it more difficult at first to communicate with the you, the regressionist. The reason for this is that this is a resting period for them as they are between lives and they are not as connected to you or interested in communicating. They are usually more interested in the feelings of peace and tranquillity they are re-experiencing.

However, it is in the Bardo state that the most in depth answers can be received and where the final healing of emotional energy takes places.

If a person has difficulty receiving information during the Bardo state then I recommend having them ask for one of their spiritual guides to come forward and assist them or for their higher self to come forward and assist them.

THE BARDO TECHNIQUE

GO THE POINT IN TIME just before your death. You are arriving there now. (pause)

Where are you?

How do you feel?

How old are you?

Do you know that you are going to die?

Is there anyone there with you, or not?

How do you feel about death?

Now very easily, you're going to move through your death and lift out of the body. It's very easy and comfortable, you're simply floating upwards now, higher and higher. (pause) Floating up, higher and higher.

Now you're going to look back down towards your body. Finding it. Noticing where you left it. (pause)

How did your body die?

Now go to your funeral, if there is one, and tell me what you notice. (pause)

You're going to move forward now, to a point where you are going to be able to examine and understand that lifetime more clearly. You're moving through space and you're arriving at that point now. You're going to be able to understand and examine that life more easily now. Just answer my questions with the very first thing that comes to mind, without judging or analyzing it.

Looking back on that lifetime, is there anything you wanted to do but were unable to do?

What was your purpose in that life?

Did you learn anything in particular in that life?

Are you carrying anything forward from that lifetime to be balanced or healed?

Are you carrying any emotions towards anyone in that lifetime?

If yes, then towards who and what are the emotions?

NOTE:

THIS IS THE TIME TO undergo the healing and releasing of any emotions that may be lingering. If the person has responded that they have lingering emotions towards someone, then tell the person to invite the higher self of that person to be there with them now. Give them a moment and then ask them if they can sense the spirit of that person.

If for some reason they cannot sense the spirit of that person, ask them if they are reluctant to release the emotions and why.

Normally, however, it is easy for the person to sense the spirit of the personality from the past. Once they have then it is time to encourage them to heal any emotions which they have held within them. It is important to tell them that they will not actually hurt the person by expressing their truth and emotions but they now have an opportunity to heal. Also tell them that they will not be judged for their emotions and that it is perfectly safe to say and express anything.

The following questions can be used to encourage that process:

What are you feeling towards that person or those people?

Were you able to express those feelings at all during the previous life?

What would you like to say to that being now?

Say it directly to the spirit and out loud?

NOTE:

IF THE PERSON IS VOICING their emotions weakly and you notice a tightness in their breathing or simply sense that they are not truly expressing themselves freely, then it can be necessary to encourage them to speak more loudly and to breathe more deeply as I discussed in the chapter on releasing energy.

Tell them that this is their only opportunity to finally release all that they have been holding and they have to take that opportunity and use it to the fullest now.

This leads to some final questions to ask in the Bardo state.

Is there anyone in that lifetime who is currently with you in your present life?

If so, who and who are they now?

BRINGING THEM BACK TO THE PRESENT

IT IS QUITE EASY TO bring someone back to the present although it must be remembered that they will often feel light-headed for a while afterwards. The technique is:

You're going to come back to the present now. I'm going to count you upwards from 1 to 10. With each number you will become stronger and more alert.

1 - coming back easily and slowly

2 - back to the present, clear headed and alert

3 - feeling yourself becoming stronger

4 - feeling your present body now

5 - your breathing is becoming stronger

6 - feeling your body wanting to move and stretch now

7 - coming back to the present, alert and refreshed

8 - fully back into the room here

9 - alert and refreshed, your breathing become strong,

10 - fully back into the room, now.

Open your eyes when you are ready and allow yourself to stretch and take some deep breaths.

NOTE:

AT THIS POINT IT IS helpful to rub the person's feet and shins as well as their hands as it is often difficult for them to start the movement of their bodies. This also creates a movement of energy in order to make them feel more grounded and alert.

After they have opened their eyes and stretched a little, encourage them to sit up very slowly as they may feel a little light-headed or dizzy. Then once they have sat for a moment, have them stand and then rub their spine up and down a few times to stimulate the flow of energy in their bodies.

Then offer the person something to drink, either some water, juice or tea while you sit and talk about the regression and piece together how the previous life has effected the present life.

Take the time with the person to ensure that they are alert and grounded before letting them go home and especially encourage them to walk a little outside and take some deep breaths before driving a vehicle.

Also tell the person how it is common that they feel shaky and ungrounded for the rest of the day and that it is wise for them to eat something soon and to rest for the remainder of the day. It is also quite common to return from a regression with a headache. This will usually go after the person has walked around outside a little and inhaled some fresh air.

Tell them that it is common for them to feel a little nauseous for the first twenty four hours, especially if they have released any old energy.

They are wise to watch their dreams for the next few days, as often they will receive more memories of that previous life during their dream states.

If the person continues to feel shaky or headachy after a few days, then it is a sign that they have more energy to release from that previous life and need to either return for another regression or try to expel the remaining energy by exercise and deep breathing as well as walks or runs in the fresh air.

Sometimes the person can expel excess energy by deeply exhaling, as though blowing a trumpet.

CHAPTER TWENTY-SEVEN

Moving Through Blocks

ONCE IN A WHILE A person has difficulty remembering one of their previous lives. This can be caused by a number of factors. The person can be nervous and simply unsure of what is going to happen and therefore they control too much and do not allow themselves to relax enough.

There can also be a block to remembering a previous life because the higher self feels the person is not yet ready to deal with the memory of a previous life. This is often the case if there is a particularly horrific lifetime which is needing to be healed, but is too overwhelming for the person to remember as yet.

In this case, it is important to remember that you cannot push someone into remembering something they are not ready for.

In the following paragraphs I give a number of ways to get around a resistant person's mind in order to unlock the past memories. However, if a person is still unable to have a past life recall, then it is a sure sign that they are not ready and they should not be forced to continue.

When someone has difficulty in remembering a previous life, discuss it with them after the session so that they understand that it is not because they are a failure, but simply because their higher self is protecting them from remembering something they are not ready to remember yet. This block to remembering can usually be eased in time and with a few exercises to assure the higher self that the person is indeed capable of dealing with any memory that may surface.

Often a block is created by fear. Fear of either the unknown or fear that they have done something horrible in a previous life or have been the victim of something horrible. If a person is unable to remember a previous life, then I encourage discussing their fears with them.

By reassuring someone that a past life memory is just that, a memory, and that by remembering even the most horrible of past lives, we are more able to have a better understanding of our present lives.

I would also explain to people that we have all been both the victimizer and the victim in previous lives. We can't all be good guys all the time. Then who would be doing all the cruel deeds. Somebody has to and that somebody is us. It is a part of the human experience to experience both the negative and the positive of human experiences. It is important to remember that they are just that - experiences. We take them on with personalities and bodies in order to learn and evolve.

Approximately one out of five people will initially have difficulty seeing a past life vision in their first regression. Most often this is because of nervousness or a need to control.

They will move through the regression technique trying to analyze everything that is being said and they will on some level, resist the relaxation of their bodies.

This can be most natural in many people as they are not used to losing control and that can be a tremendous fear to their minds. This is why it is helpful during the technique to stress that they are actually, still in control, but relaxed.

During the regression, a controller will find themselves analyzing every step of the way or trying to change it in some way. I had a case of a man who when we got to the door in the time tunnel, he started creating numerous doors, always changing. From the door to his house, to the door to my house, to many other doors. Also during the relaxation part, he kept changing the elevator into elevators he had known. This is a way of controlling and not feeling the body relaxing.

Again, it is important to stress during the regression the need to feel the body, rather than think about the words being spoken.

What happens in these instances is that the person gets through the doorway and nothing happens. They do not see or sense anything and they simply feel the same as did when they laid on the bed. They may be a little more relaxed but not enough to be in a Theta state.

The first thing to do in this instance, is to relax the person more. This is done by having the person then create an image of steps moving down into the earth. Tell them that the steps are vague and that they needn't focus on them, but rather, to feel themselves walking down the steps as you count them down from eight to one.

Then count them down slowly, with each number having them feel themselves stepping down, going deeper within. Stepping down and relaxing even more.

When they reach the bottom, then it is necessary to recreate moving through the time tunnel, only this time eliminate the door and simply create an opening, such as a doorway.

I eliminate the door in order to take away any opportunity for the person's mind to hang onto an image and analyze it.

I reiterate to the person that the time tunnel is dark and vague and so there is nothing for them to really see at all. Rather they are to feel themselves moving through the tunnel and back through time until they arrive at the doorway and then they will move through the doorway and into the body.

Then you begin again to have the person look at their feet and then their body.

If there is still no connection to a body, I would ask the person the following questions:

1. What are you feeling now?
2. What is it like around you?
3. Do you sense any colors, or just blackness?
4. Do you feel as though you are floating or standing or what?

It often surprises people to find that even though they do not feel as though they are in a body, suddenly when asked how they are feeling, they feel fear, for instance. This is an important clue which means they are afraid to get into the body for some reason, and you need to find out what that reason is by asking the person what they are afraid of.

When someone is unable to sense or see anything at this point, it takes experience on the regressionist's part in being a detective. Usually the subconscious will give clues as to what the problem is and you need to find those clues by asking the right questions, such as, "What do you feel?"

If no obvious clues are given then I move to the next step.

Once in a while a person will move into a regression and arrive in between lives, whereby they are simply floating, with no attachment to feelings of any kind. When this is the case it is necessary to reconnect the person with their most recent life by having them look for the earth and then move towards it.

TECHNIQUE FOR BLOCK

You're going to look now for the planet earth. It's there somewhere, I want you to find it now. (pause)

Finding the earth now and you're going to feel yourself being pulled towards it, getting closer and closer now. Being pulled towards the planet and now towards some land.

You're getting closer now to some land, somewhere on the planet. It's there and your going to sense it and see it now.

Noticing the land, noticing if there are trees, sand, hills, or whatever. Looking at the land.

Now you're going to notice someone is there on the land, a person. You're going to sense and see them now. Finding them and noticing them. There's someone there. Find them and look at them now. (pause)

Noticing that person below you and noticing how big the person is. Tell me now how big or little the person is?

Tell me now is the person a male or female?

What is the person wearing?

What is the person doing?

Is there anyone else around, or not?

How does the person seem to you, happy or not, or something else?

Now at the count of three you're going to feel yourself being pulled into the body of that person. One, (pause) two, (pause) and three, being pulled into the body.

Now you're going to look around you, you're in the body now and you're going to awaken your feelings and senses from inside the body now.

END

Now you begin to ask the same type of questions which were stated in the regression technique. Although, normally I would simply go with the moment and ask the person, "What is happening next?" and continue asking that.

Sometimes when regressing someone there is simply a resistance to entering the body and by giving them a look first from a distance they are usually more willing then to get into the body.

However, they can watch the lifetime from a distance if they prefer it. This is common for those who feel it may be too intense to get into the body. Never push someone to enter the previous body, but encourage it, because it is much more real for them when they are in the body.

If they simply watch the lifetime from a distance, then they will be more likely to think afterwards that they could have made it up. The reason is simply because they did not have the emotional connection with the previous life when they watched it from above, nor did they feel the physical difference of being in a different body.

Sometimes when I notice a resistance in someone I will encourage them to watch the past life from their higher self's perspective at the beginning, which is what one is doing when they see the memory from above/outside, but then to enter the body later when they become more comfortable with the situation. This will ensure a more intense emotional connection and they will not be able to refute the reality of the experience afterwards.

I have heard of therapists simply having people see various lifetimes passing by during the regression. I do not feel that this is a true regression. It is a memory but the person is not actually connecting with the previous lives and cannot see themselves from the front. They can only see themselves from a distance and from behind, which is the higher self's perspective.

The only way you can see your face in a regression is to look in a mirrored surface whilst in the body itself.

This leads me to explain why so many people think they are someone famous in a previous life like Cleopatra and Napoleon. If I could count how many Cleopatra and Napoleon wannabe's there were I would be overwhelmed.

As many regressionists simply flip people through images of their past lives, they miss the truth of the experience.

For instance, if a person is simply experiencing lifetimes passing by in quick but brief, images, they are not connecting with the bodies that they are in and are simply remembering things that they have seen.

An example is a client named Peter. I regressed him into a previous life and he explained to me rather quickly, before looking down at his own body and feet, that someone was in front of him kneeling. He explained to me that the man in front of him kneeling was wearing very beautiful clothes with ornate silk and brocade fabric. He then stated to me that the man was greeting him with the words, my lord, Louis XIV.

The man then gleefully told me that he was Louis XIV.

I replied that that was indeed fine, but I would like to get some more detail about what was going on around him. I asked him to look around him to his right. He did and responded that the people to his right were also bowing to him. I then asked him to look to his left and tell me if there was anything there to see.

He then looked to his left and I noticed his eyebrows suddenly squeeze together. I asked him what he was seeing and he replied in a rather annoyed tone, "Oh, he's Louis XIV, sitting beside me. I'm standing beside him."

I then asked him to please look down at his own body and to feel his body and tell me what he experienced. He told me that he was actually a lackee standing beside the king holding some sort of flagpole.

So much for being Louis XIV. However, it is a common mistake which people make in regressions when they flip through them quickly and do not spend the time looking at their own body and of those around them.

The reason so many people think they are Cleopatra and Napoleon is because that is who they are seeing when they first enter the regression. They are in the body looking at their queen or their emperor and the reason the queen or emperor has come up first in the regression is because it was such a high point in their previous life to see their queen or emperor, that

that is the first thing that is remembered. It was an important point in their life as it is for many who see their leader up close.

This is why it is necessary to look closely at oneself first before getting caught up in what is happening in front of them or around them. So many people think they are Cleopatra and Napoleon because so many people saw them in their past lives and will remember it.

If after having a person come closer to their previous lives through first finding the earth and then finding themselves on the earth, they still don't see or sense anything, then it is time to connect with their higher self and receive some answers. This is done by first creating an ancient book into one's inner vision which will help in receiving answers from a higher source.

THE TECHNIQUE

I WOULD LIKE YOU NOW to create in your mind an image of a very ancient book. This book is actually called the Akashic Records Book. It has all of the records of your previous lives as well as your present. It is going to look very old and large. I want you to bring that book now into your inner vision. Tell me when you can see it. (pause and wait for a yes reply).

The way this book works is simple. You ask it a question, then turn the page and the answer is then on the next page.

So first I would like you to feel yourself open the book and you will simply notice a blank page. (pause)

Now I would like you to ask the book the following question, then turn the page and see the answer on the next page.

Am I ready to remember my previous lives? (pause)
Turn the page and see the answer now. It's there. (pause)
Tell me what it says, yes or no.

END

THE QUESTIONS YOU THEN CHOOSE to ask the Book of Akashic Records is dependent on the answer you have just received. If the answer is a yes that the person is ready to see the previous lives, then you would ask the book, "Why am I unable to see my previous lives?" as well you can ask, "Do I have any fears or blocks to remembering my previous lives?" and "What can I do to remember my previous lives?"

The book will then give the answers which will help you to discover what the person's blocks really are and what needs to be done next.

Sometimes there is no block, simply resistance, to which there is one more thing which can be done with the book's help.

You would have the person ask the book to show them a picture of their previous life, then have them turn the page and see a picture of the previous life.

If they can see a picture of the previous life, then I would have them describe it to me and then tell them that the picture is going to begin to move, like a movie and they can watch it from a distance. Then again they can see what the person in the picture is doing and possibly, get into the body as they become more familiar with it and with the life from a distance.

The previous techniques are most helpful for those who are resistant or controlling and find it difficult to see or remember anything in a previous life.

CHAPTER TWENTY-EIGHT

Awakening Inner Vision

IF SOMEONE IS UNABLE TO have any visual experiences during a regression, then it is necessary to have them undertake some exercises to awaken their inner vision. These, if practiced daily, will usually take only a few weeks before the person is then ready to undergo another regression.

The first exercise is to create a quiet space to relax where the lights are not too bright and to close their eyes and picture their present home. Then to picture their childhood home.

After one has created the visual memory of one's childhood home, then it is helpful to go through the home and look for details, including colors of walls, kitchen floors, cupboards and bedspreads, etc. Go through the house and look at paintings and wall coverings as well.

Doing this exercise daily will help to stimulate the inner vision and by the end of two weeks the inner vision is usually much stronger and more vivid.

Then the person needs to learn how to relax into an Alpha or Theta state. To do this they need to have a tape recording of a relaxation technique, which is similar to the beginning of the regression technique.

This can easily be created by the person by making a recording themselves and then placing it beside them as they lay on their bed.

It is important in awakening inner vision that the person be relaxed enough to be in a deep Alpha or a light Theta state. By regularly practicing their relaxation techniques with the help of a taped recording, it will not be long, probably a few weeks, before they are ready to be regressed again.

Often people have telephoned me after practicing the relaxation only a few days and expressed how they were already getting glimpses of past life memories starting to surface.

Another avenue to assist in awakening the inner vision is to practice meditation. Not the form of meditation where you are visualizing something, as that is not really meditation at all, but rather to simply sit and become aware of your breathing and body.

Courses on meditation are always helpful in getting a person to move into deeper states of relaxation, including a Theta awareness, which is often the most difficult thing for those who have not been able to remember previous lives.

Chapter Twenty-Nine

Regressing Yourself

Regressing yourself can be easy enough, but it must be remembered that in the beginning, unless you are an experienced meditator, it will be difficult to sustain the regression because you will most likely either fall asleep or be unable to move yourself forward through the life.

To regress yourself, I recommend making a tape recording of the regression technique and laying it beside you while you lay down and relax.

In making the regression tape, you will only be able to take it so far. That is you can state on the recording that you have moved through the doorway and into the body and you can even then ask on the tape for you to look down at your feet and then up your body. From there, however, you become restricted at what you can say on the tape. This is what I recommend.

After asking yourself to look at your body, then ask to look around you and to see where you are. Then it is necessary to create a pause long enough on the recording to allow you the opportunity to see around you.

Next ask to go find your home and family and again leave enough time, approximately one minute for you to do so.

After this, I would recommend asking yourself to go through your day and find out what you do on a typical day.

From there it is quite difficult to continue asking specific questions on a taped recording and I simply recommend that approximately every minute or so to ask, "What's happening next."

This statement will encourage you, while in the regression, to continue to move through the life. Otherwise without that encouragement, you will likely find yourself stuck in one area of the life and unable to move forward.

Eventually, you will either fall asleep or drift back to the present. However, once you have moved through a number of self regressions, you will find it easier to move yourself through the life as you will master having the awareness of both the previous life and the present enough to keep yourself moving.

This type of self regression is often not as deep as one undertaken with a therapist. The reason for this is that with a therapist you are more able to let yourself move deeper, whereas when you are doing a self regression, you need to maintain an awareness of your present self enough so as to help move you through the regression.

With practice, however, self regressions can become just as intense as with a therapist.

If you come across a lifetime while doing a self regression that seems too emotionally intense for you to deal with on your own, then I recommend coming back to the present and waiting until you can have someone assist you.

To come back from a self-regression takes a little longer than when assisted. You will find yourself drifting from the regression because it will be difficult to hold it without someone encouraging you. When you drift from the vision focus on your breathing and your present body and you will soon feel completely alert and present again. However, it may take a little longer for you to feel strong and grounded and I recommend deep breathing for a few minutes and rubbing your legs and feet as soon as you are able to move freely.

CHAPTER THIRTY

Finding A Regression Therapist

MANY PEOPLE CONTINUALLY ASK ME how to find a good regression therapist and I recommend asking some basic questions over the telephone before going to an actual regression. These are the following:

1. How long do you spend in a session and how many lives do you go through in one session? (It should take approximately 1 1/2 hours to go through one or maybe two lives, if the first is difficult to sense.)
2. Do you take people in the Bardo state or Astral state? (If they don't, then find someone else.)
3. Do you work with energy? (It is vital that the regression therapist be able to help you release energy that may be blocked in your body or be triggered during a traumatic memory.)
4. How do you heal or balance the past blocks and karmas? (The therapist should bring higher selves forward in order that you be able to express freely any unresolved issues. They should also encourage deep breathing and sound release.)
5. Do you do the regression in your home or in an office? (A home is preferable although an office with sound- proofing and a place to lie down is fine.)

6. What do you do if I go into uncontrollable teeth chattering and shaking all over? (The therapist should help you to emit the blocked energy, not to try to calm you down.)

The above are some basic questions to ask a regression therapist over the phone before making an appointment for a regression.

It is also helpful to ask if they have had much experience with traumatic lives and blocked energy. This will help you to know if you are going to a therapist with experience in intense regression work, not simply a therapist who skips you through visual memories for entertainment purposes.

About the Author

Laurel Phelan is an expert in the field of reincarnation and regression therapy. She has taught psychologists and therapists in England, Canada and the USA. As the Author of Guinevere, she first shared her experiences of reincarnation and regression therapy in 1996. As a regression therapist for 25 years who has helped over 2,000 people around the world, she is a unique expert in the field of both reincarnation and hypnosis.

LaVergne, TN USA
22 March 2010
176811LV00001B/177/P